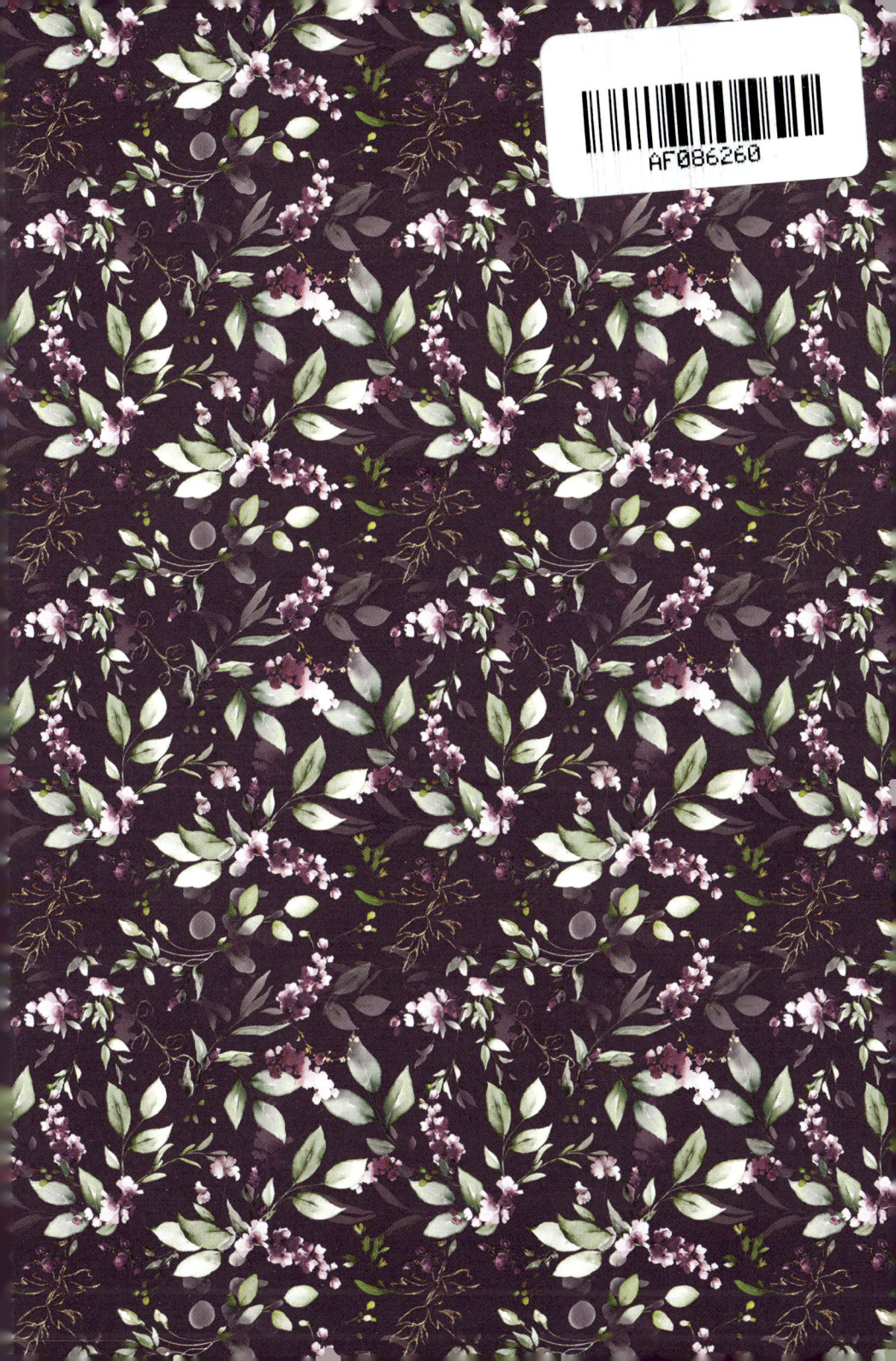

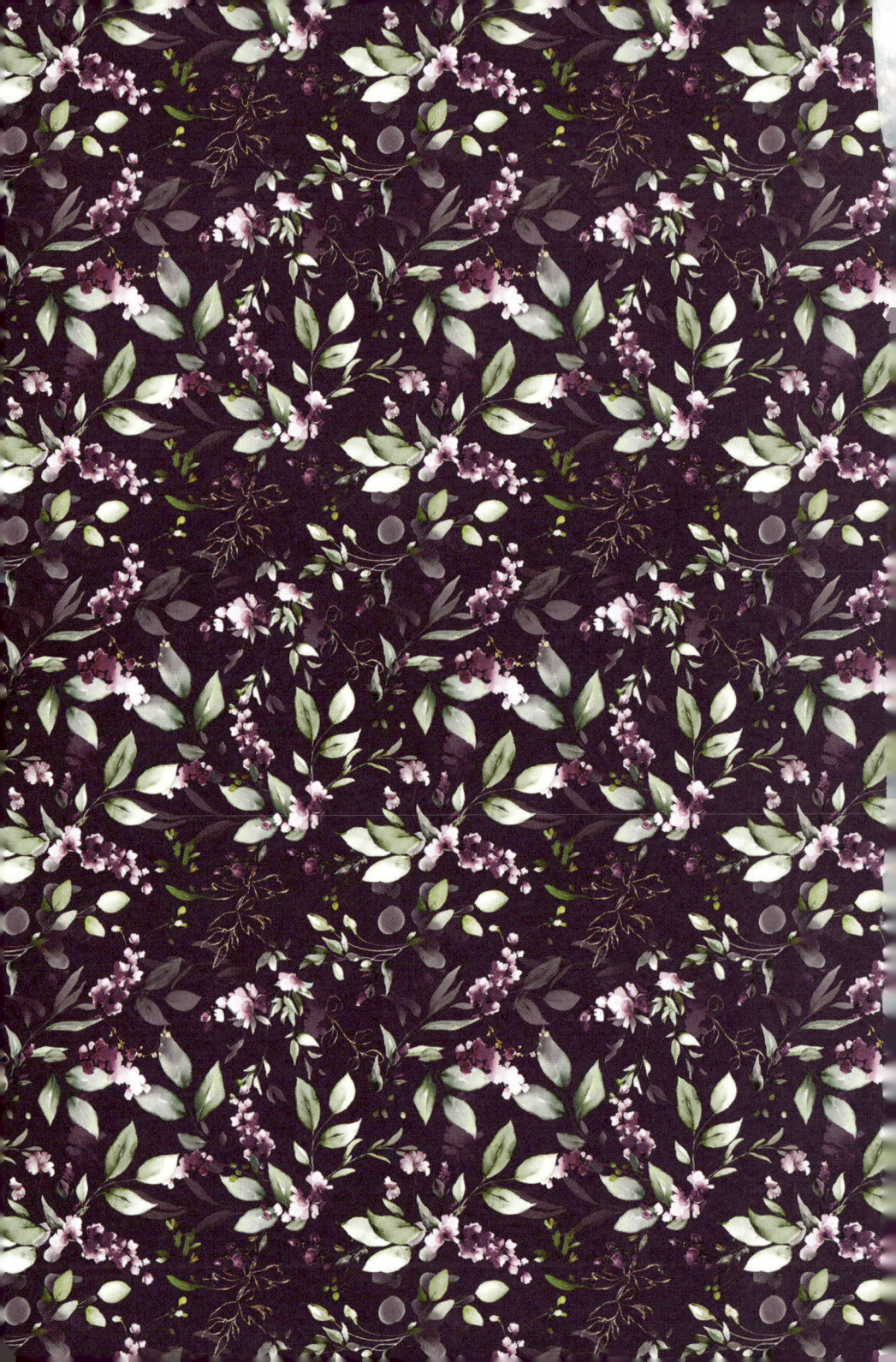

The Nurturing Power of Aromatherapy

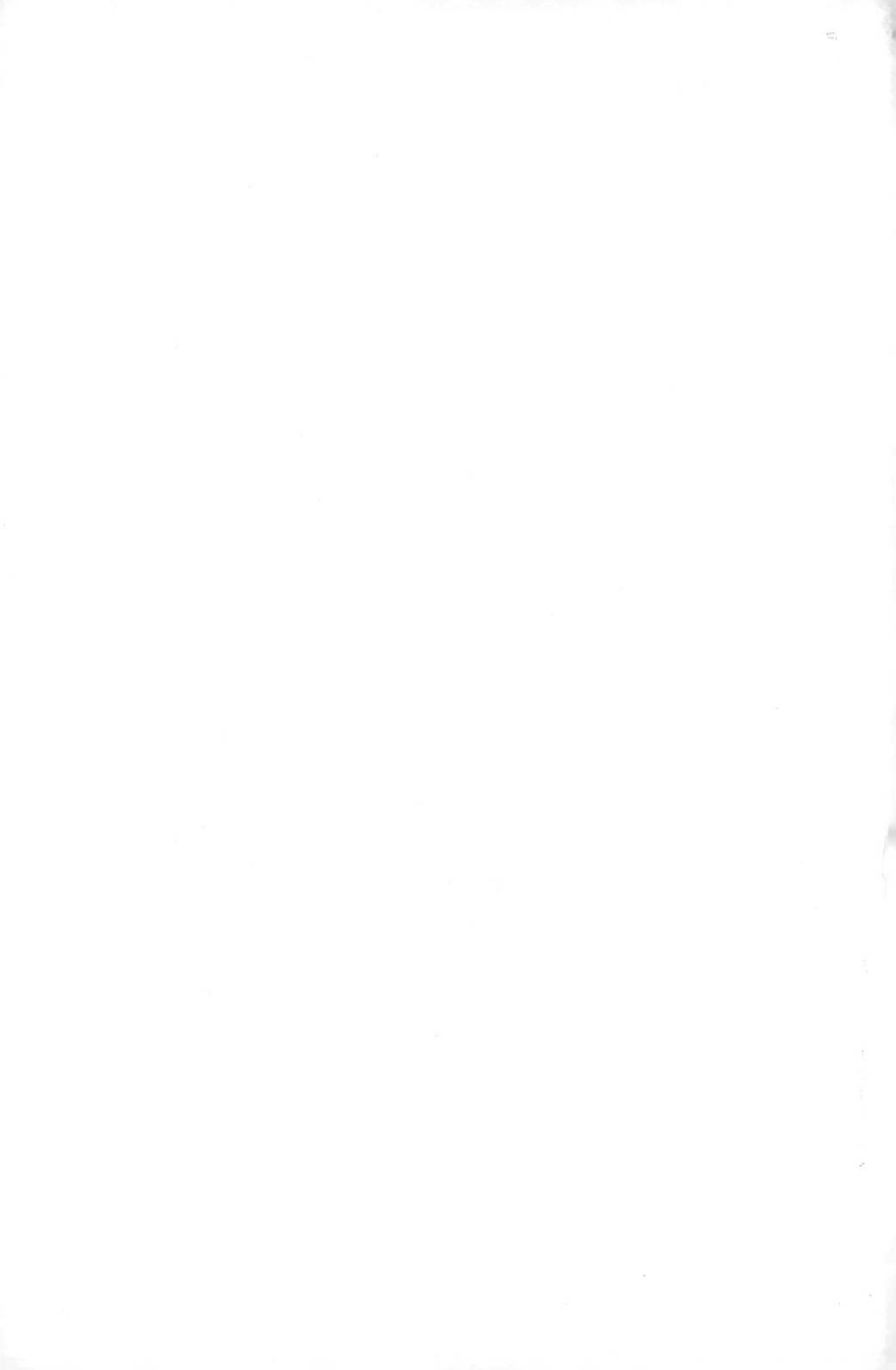

The Nurturing Power of Aromatherapy

A practical guide to essential oils and its uses

NIRMAL MINAWALA

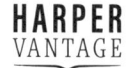

HarperCollins *Publishers* India

First published in India by HarperVantage 2025
An imprint of HarperCollins *Publishers*
HarperCollins *Publishers* India, Cyber City,
Building 10-A, Gurugram, Haryana – 122002, India
www.harpercollins.co.in

2 4 6 8 10 9 7 5 3 1

Copyright © Nirmal Minawala

P-ISBN: 978-93-6213-049-5
E-ISBN: 978-93-6213-065-5

This book's content is for general educational purposes only and does not constitute or substitute for professional medical advice, diagnosis, or treatment. Consult a medical professional before using essential oils or remedies, especially if you have medical conditions, are pregnant, nursing, or on medication. The quality and application of essential oils are beyond the author's and publisher's control, and no responsibility is accepted. The author and publisher make no warranties about the suitability, safety or effectiveness of the described methods or products and are not liable for any loss, damage, or injury from their use or misuse.

Nirmal Minawala asserts the moral right
to be identified as the author of this work.

All rights reserved. No part of this publication may be reproduced,
stored in a retrieval system, or transmitted, in any form or by any means,
electronic, mechanical, photocopying, recording or otherwise,
without the prior permission of the publishers.

Without limiting the exclusive rights of any author, contributor or the publisher of this publication, any unauthorized use of this publication to train generative artificial intelligence (AI) technologies is expressly prohibited. HarperCollins also exercise their rights under Article 4(3) of the Digital Single Market Directive 2019/790 and expressly reserve this publication from the text and data-mining exception.

Typeset in Arno Pro
by HarperCollins *Publishers* India Pvt. Ltd

Printed and bound at
Thomson Press (India) Ltd

*

HarperCollins *Publishers*, Macken House, 39/40 Mayor Street Upper, Dublin 1,
D01 C9W8, Ireland

Table of Contents

Foreword   6

Author's Note   7

Introduction - My Fragrant Journey   8

Chapter 1 - What is Aromatherapy?   11

Chapter 2 - Holistic Approach   17

Chapter 3 - Extraction of Essential Oils   21

Chapter 4 - Simple and Effective Methods of Using Essential Oils   25

Chapter 5 - Types of Essential Oils   31

Chapter 6 - Carrier or Base Oils   101

Chapter 7 - Aromatherapy and Skincare   109

Chapter 8 - Aromatherapy and Emotions   113

Chapter 9 - Aromatherapy and Chakras   127

Chapter 10 - Perfumery   141

Chapter 11 - Aromatherapy Blend Formulas   147

Chapter 12 - Therapeutic Index For Some Common Problems   159

Foreword

I am pleased to introduce Aroma Treasures, a pioneering force in India's aromatherapy landscape. Founded by Mr Nirmal Minawala and Mrs Aradhana Minawala, this esteemed brand has been transforming lives since 2000. Through their commitment to natural ingredients and innovative products, Aroma Treasures has established itself as a beacon of excellence. Mr Minawala's previous book, *Aromatherapy Made Easy*, and his presentation series on Astha Channel have empowered thousands. Through their visionary leadership, they have created a brand that seamlessly blends beauty, nature, and science. Let us draw inspiration from their remarkable story and embark on a path towards a healthier, more harmonious life.

– **Jawed Habib**

Author's Note

This book is an extension of a one Aradhana and I wrote twenty five years ago, *Aromatherapy Made Easy*. We combined all our knowledge along with wonderful references from books by Shirley Price, Valerie Ann Worwood and others.

Today, as I complete this extension, I'm ever grateful to my best friend and partner, my wife. Our journey nurturing our company, Aroma Treasures, together has been has been a rollercoaster ride with many amazing moments. Though she is no longer with us in the physical form, I will always cherish the wonderful time we spent together.

My fragrant journey is a part of my spiritual journey blessed by my gurus, and I am ever grateful to them for the immense love, guidance, and blessings they have graced us with. As I look at myself today, I am blessed with all the fragrances and colours of life. There is total fulfilment and contentment with the abundance life has showered upon us. If life did not give us something, it compensated us with something better. If it took away something, it replaced the space with joy and peace. What more could I ask for? I always felt like a privileged child of God, being taken through the best school of life and made to blossom into a beautiful flower.

I want to express my gratitude to my family and friends, who have supported me throughout my journey on this planet. I am also grateful to my friend and editor, Varsha Naik, for helping me make this book a reality.

Introduction

My Fragrant Journey:

Going down memory lane, it feels like the universe had a hand in guiding and nudging me in a particular direction. Somewhat unknowingly, that path has led me to where I am today, with the most wonderful people around me. We often hear that only good luck brings you to the right place at the right time. I couldn't agree more and would like to add that luck can be generated by sowing the right seeds in life.

During my college years, I had the unique opportunity to immerse myself in a well-equipped fragrance laboratory, where I delved into the world of natural and synthetic materials from across the globe. This experience allowed me to experiment with the most unconventional ideas in blending fragrances for the cosmetic and agarbatti industries, setting the stage for my journey through diverse branches of alternative systems of medicine and healing. Homoeopathy, Bach Flower Remedies, Magnet Therapy, Pendulum Dowsing, Pyramid Power, Herbal Remedies, Hatha Yoga, Heal Your Life by Louise Hay and Mindfulness Meditation were some of the different systems I dabbled in. I found that applying a combination of these techniques offered relief for some of the issues people came to me with. But working with natural essential oils, understanding and using them to help people, has come the easiest to me.

I am grateful to nature for giving me opportunities that served as challenges and for guiding me to formulate different blends of essential oils to treat the many issues I've encountered over the years. I would often ask friends or family if they had any physical or emotional issues, research those discomforts and make oil blends for them. Over time, we were able to develop blends to resolve issues such as sinusitis, gas and cramps, muscular and joint pain, sleep disorders, mood swings, PMS, migraine, acne and skin disorders; bringing relief to scores of people.

As no schools were teaching Aromatherapy in India at the time and with no means for formal training, essential oils took over my life, organically teaching me everything required to turn my passion into a profession. The oils enticed me with their exotic fragrances, extracted from peels of fruits, leaves, roots, wood, and hypnotising flowers. I fell in love with all the oils. After all, any kind of smell in the environment is just a fragrance, without judgement of being bad or good.

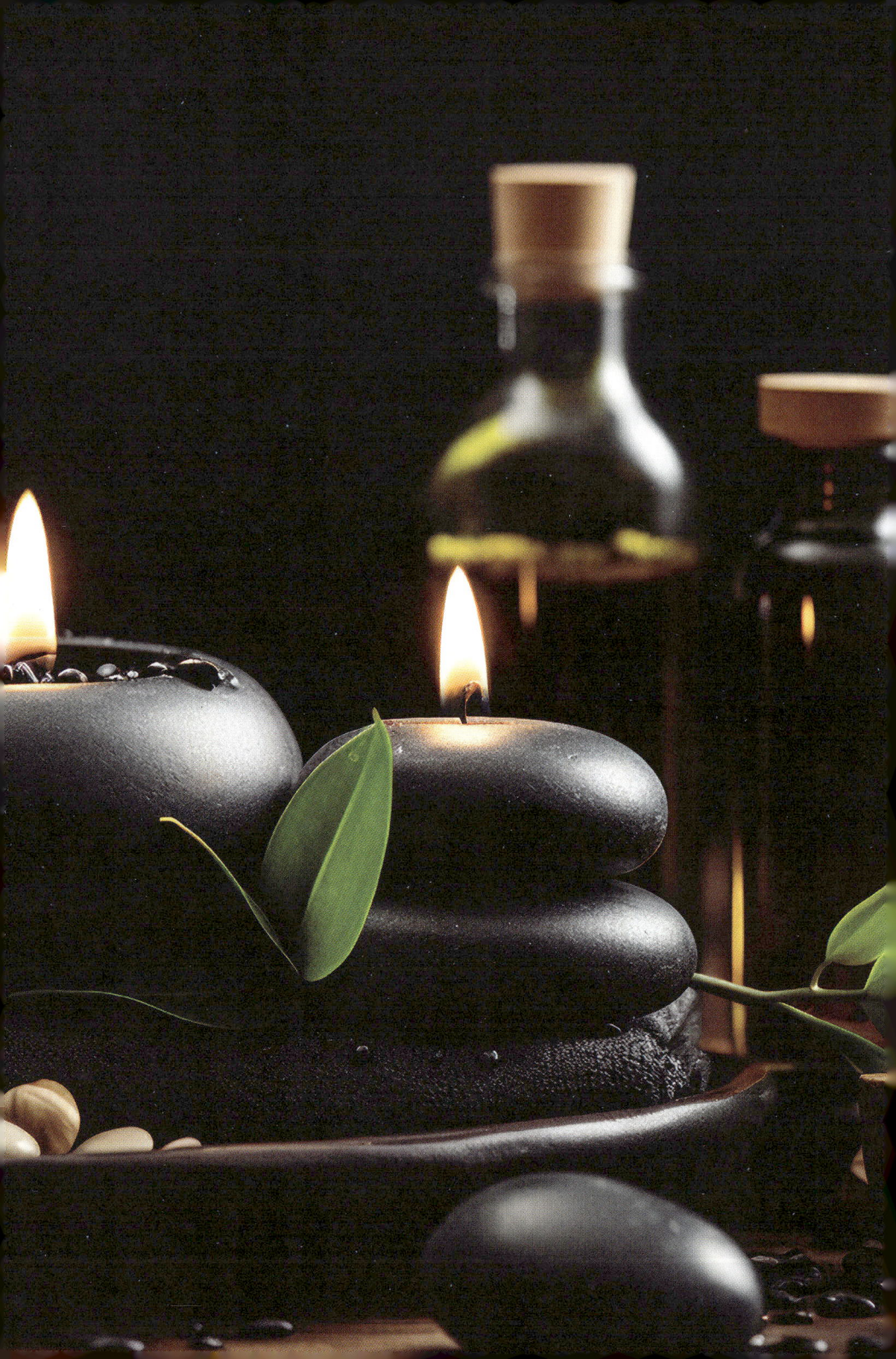

Chapter 1

What is Aromatherapy?

In our daily lives, we often overlook the potential of our sense of smell. Visual and auditory stimuli dominate our environment, from screens to sounds, leaving smell underappreciated. However, our sense of smell is the most underutilised of all our senses, yet it holds remarkable power in influencing our emotions, memories, and overall well-being.

The smell of the earth at the onset of the much-awaited rains is a divine fragrance that no perfumer in the world can duplicate. The true experience of delicious food involves indulging with the eyes and the nose. Just imagine how humdrum your taste buds would be without aroma. You may not enjoy your meal, however tasty it may be. Your nose and sense of smell predominantly determine the taste of food.

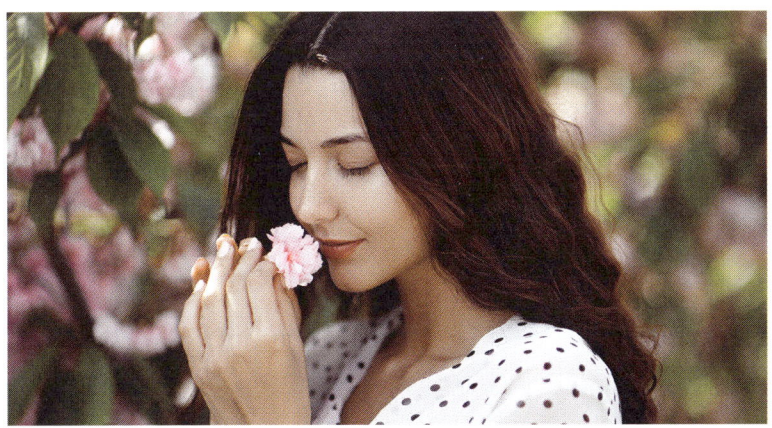

What is Aromatherapy?

The quintessential asset of smell enables us to enjoy all the wonderful fragrant plant material surrounding us, the most enchanting of them being being flowers. The aroma of flowers holds the ability to change your mood instantly. Whenever you feel troubled due to stress, worry, fear or anger, pick up a flower with a natural aroma, close your eyes and smell it. This will undoubtedly elevate your state of mind.

This happens because what you like is required to balance your mind.

Aromatherapy is an alluring journey into an ancient holistic healing art, a transformative experience that means "therapy using aromas". The aroma of a plant is released through its volatile molecules, which also carry its therapeutic value. Man recognized this property long ago and invented methods to capture this aroma to enjoy it in the future. Methods such as effleurages, steam distillation, maceration or infusion were used for different plants. The term "aromatherapy" was coined in the 20th century, but the aroma and therapeutic power of flowers and plants have been captured and used to enhance well-being for many years before that.

Attars, or ittars as they are commonly called, are perfect examples of the ancient Indian perfume industry. As chemicals did not exist in those times, perfumes were made with natural oils extracted from different parts of various plants. Attars of gulab (rose), chameli (jasmine), mogra, rajnigandha (tuberose), champak and kewda were infused in sandalwood oil and named accordingly. Many other attars, such as hina and amber, were blended only with pure essential oils.

Sandalwood oil was used as a base because of its sweetness and power to retain the aroma of anything infused in it for a very long time. Indian sandalwood oil

What is Aromatherapy?

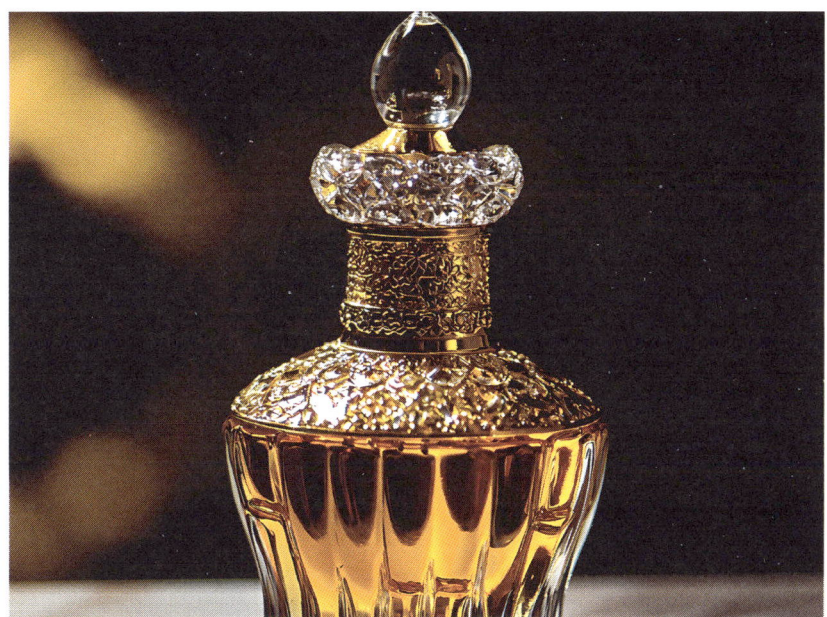

is reputed to be the best among all its cousins from around the world. The attar trend faded over time as the cost of sandalwood oil and flowers kept rising, making them unaffordable for most people. This paved the way for synthetics to emerge and dilute the charm of this wonderful ancient science.

However, since synthetic perfumes could never supersede the exotic aroma, healing, soothing and balancing properties of pure and natural essential oils, people have reverted to using them again.

Humankind have been using this therapeutic property of plants in a very convenient form: essential oils. These oils are so potent and concentrated that sometimes, you may need to distil 100 grams of plant material to get a drop of oil. Essential oils are extracted from various parts of plants, shrubs, and trees and used in different treatments to attain balance in physical, mental, and spiritual health. Because they draw from the immune systems of plants and contain antiseptic, antibiotic, antiviral, anti-inflammatory and many other medicinal properties, they help in healing, relieving and eliminating skin and health problems and soothe emotions to promote happy and healthy living.

During epidemics, plant material such as juniper was burnt, and people carried it around to protect themselves from infection. Rishis always use fragrant materials in the fire ritual known as havan or cuthoma to connect with their deities. In the animal kingdom, the power of body-emitting aromas is used to attract mates.

The body has a self-healing mechanism that takes its own time to heal and often only needs gentle stimulation of a natural product (in this case, essential oils) and an appropriate lifestyle to encourage it back to health. Essential oils enter through the bloodstream and are carried to every cell in the body, where they offer psychological and physical benefits, promoting cellular health, balance and regeneration. The aroma stimulates the brain to trigger a positive effect, and natural components of the essential oil, when drawn into the body, produce physical benefits.

In the last few decades, aromatherapy has seen a revival, and the use of essential oils has become widely popular in many countries. The demand for pure oils, regardless of their cost, has revived the extraction and availability of these natural gifts of nature. For a relaxing experience, you can add a few drops of lavender oil to your bath or use tea tree oil as a natural disinfectant for household cleaning. These are just a few examples of how essential oils can be incorporated into your daily routine.

What is Aromatherapy?

Here are some common properties of essential oils:

- Antibacterial, antimicrobic, anti-virus\ and antiseptic.
- Detoxifies: removes waste material from our bloodstream.
- Oxygenates: as oxygen is added, it stimulates the tissues.
- Gets rid of excess fluids from tissues.
- Easily absorbed by the skin because they are lipo solvents.
- They dissolve in fats.
- They dissolve in the fatty part of the skin and quickly penetrate different skin layers before entering the bloodstream. (Sebaceous glands produce sebum, which blends with the oil and makes absorption easy).
- Has the power to heal rapidly. Helps balance the nervous system.
- Promotes new cell growth and sheds dead skin cells.
- Improves circulation by regulating the action of capillaries.
- Regulates and balances body functions.
- Rehydrates for over three to six hours. Restores vitality to tissues.
- Soluble in pure alcohol, vegetable oils, and to a small extent, water.
- Volatile: when exposed to air, it evaporates quickly.
- Watery and does not leave any oily marks on paper.

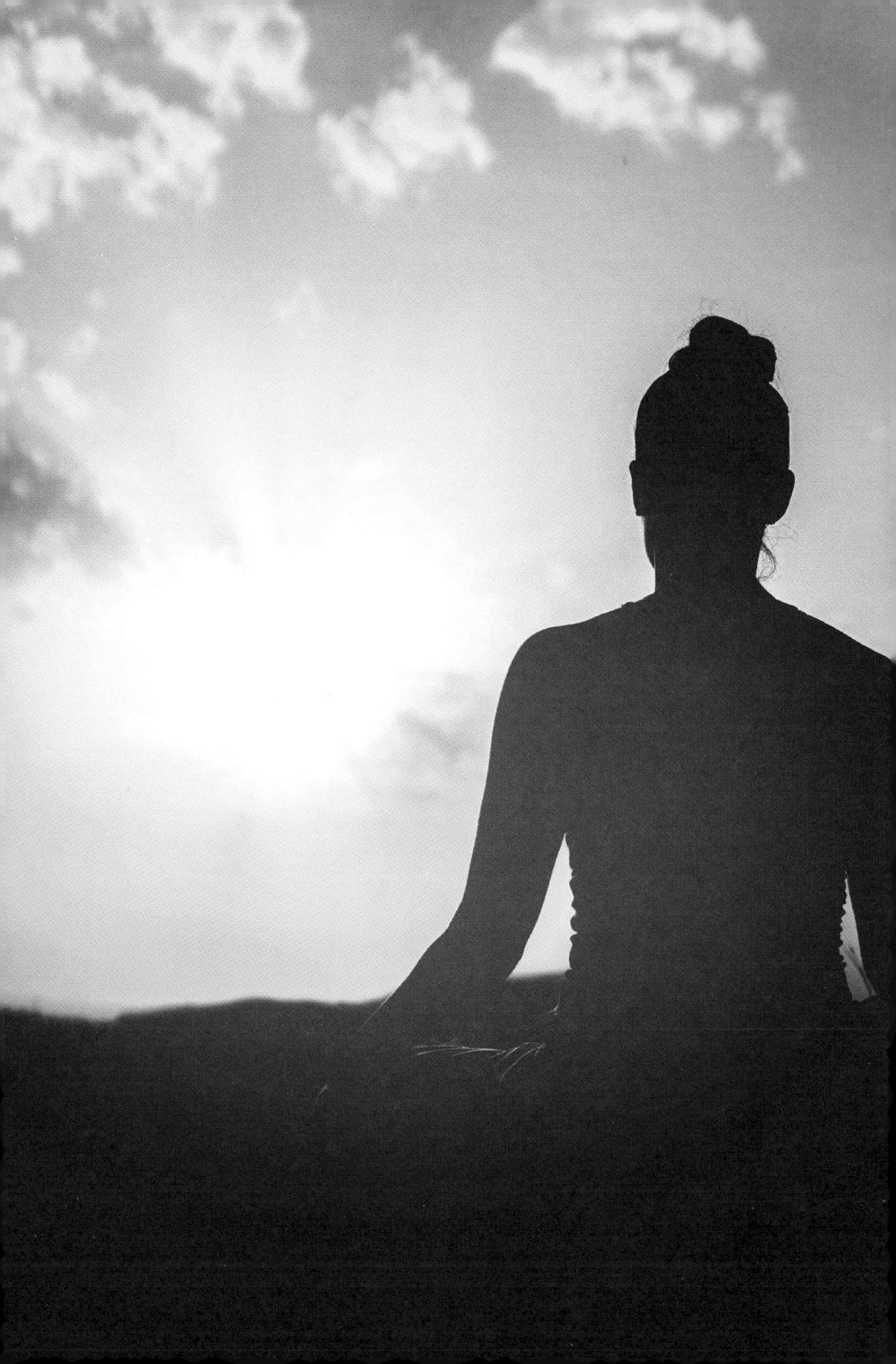

Chapter 2
Holistic Approach

Our body is a delicate instrument and will perform wonderfully if the right balance is maintained. This delicate balancing act is represented in the body's Ph level, i.e., its acid/alkaline balance. In perfect health, the alkaline level is much higher. However, pollutants, stress and a poor diet will tip the balance, increasing acid levels. As much as possible, your food intake should contain fresh foods with minimum cooking, such as fruits and vegetables. One must avoid synthetic additives, preservatives and sweets.

Water intake should be adequate throughout the day; always in its natural form (not squashes, bottled drinks, tea or coffee). Water is also a cleanser, flushing toxins from the body, leading to clear, healthy skin and helping it glow.

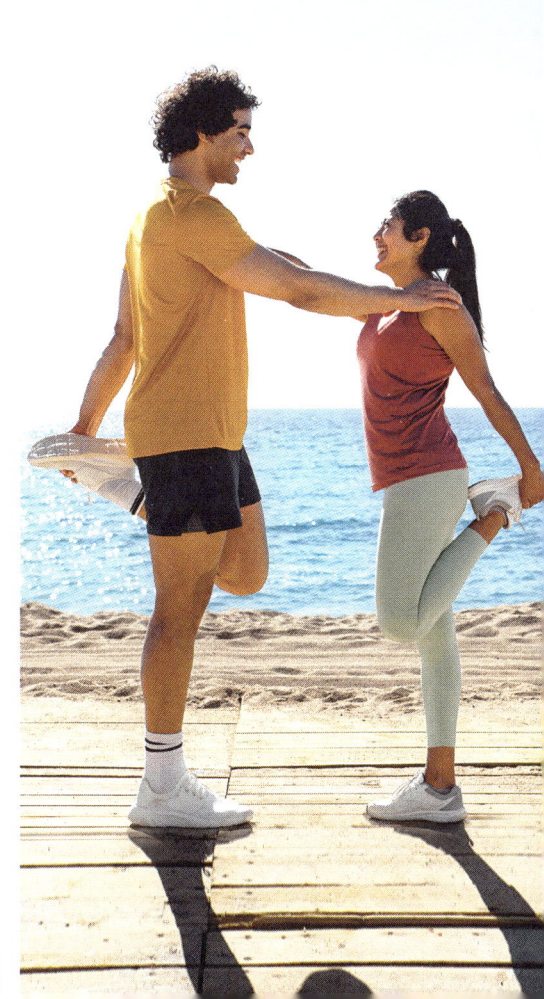

Holistic Approach

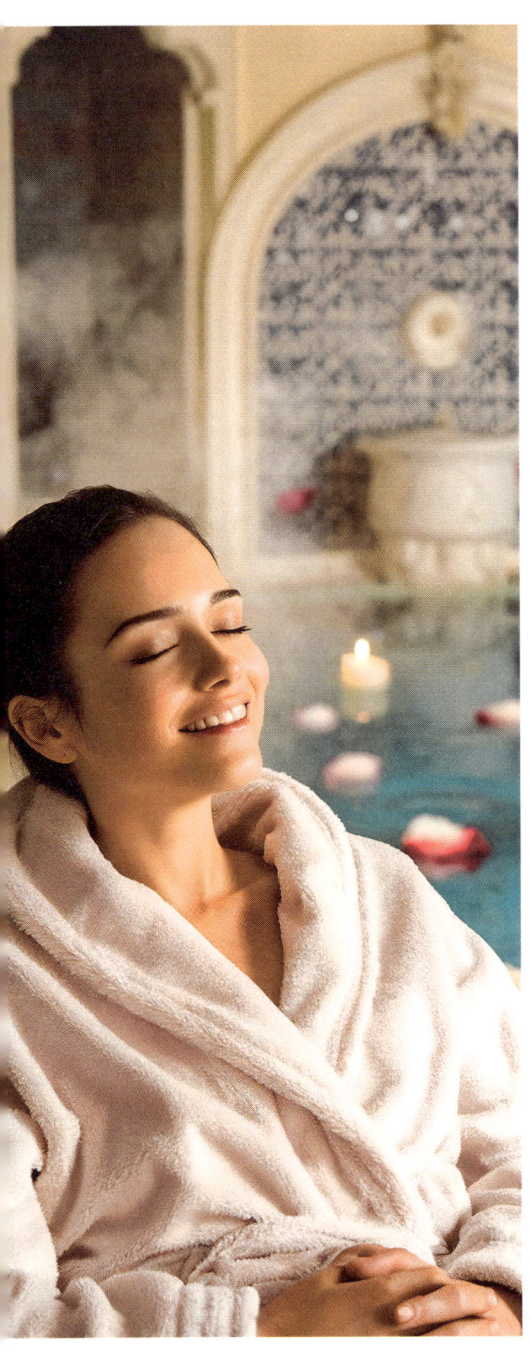

Exercise should be a regular part of your day. It helps you breathe deeply into the abdomen, giving the cells an ample supply of oxygen, which helps build up our cells and tissue growth.

Rest and sleep are critical factors in our lives. During sleep, our body repairs tissue and builds our immune system, which helps fight viruses and bacteria that attack us. Rest is another way of recharging tired tissues and relaxing tired nerves. We often overwork our bodies, resulting in stress and other diseases. It is essential to give the body a break, especially when one is sick.

Keeping stress levels under control is very important for your body. Stress could lead to a chain reaction of problems, starting with insomnia, headache, constipation, depression, anger, and stomach-related diseases. Using oils in inhalation, diffuser, bath, massage,

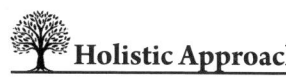 **Holistic Approach**

etc., can greatly help as it relieves stress by relaxing and calming one's mind and muscles. Natural oils are uplifting and have stimulating properties that help in getting rid of all unnecessary tensions. Oils also help induce sleep by calming and relaxing the mind and body. Good sleep is essential and one of the best ways to relieve stress.

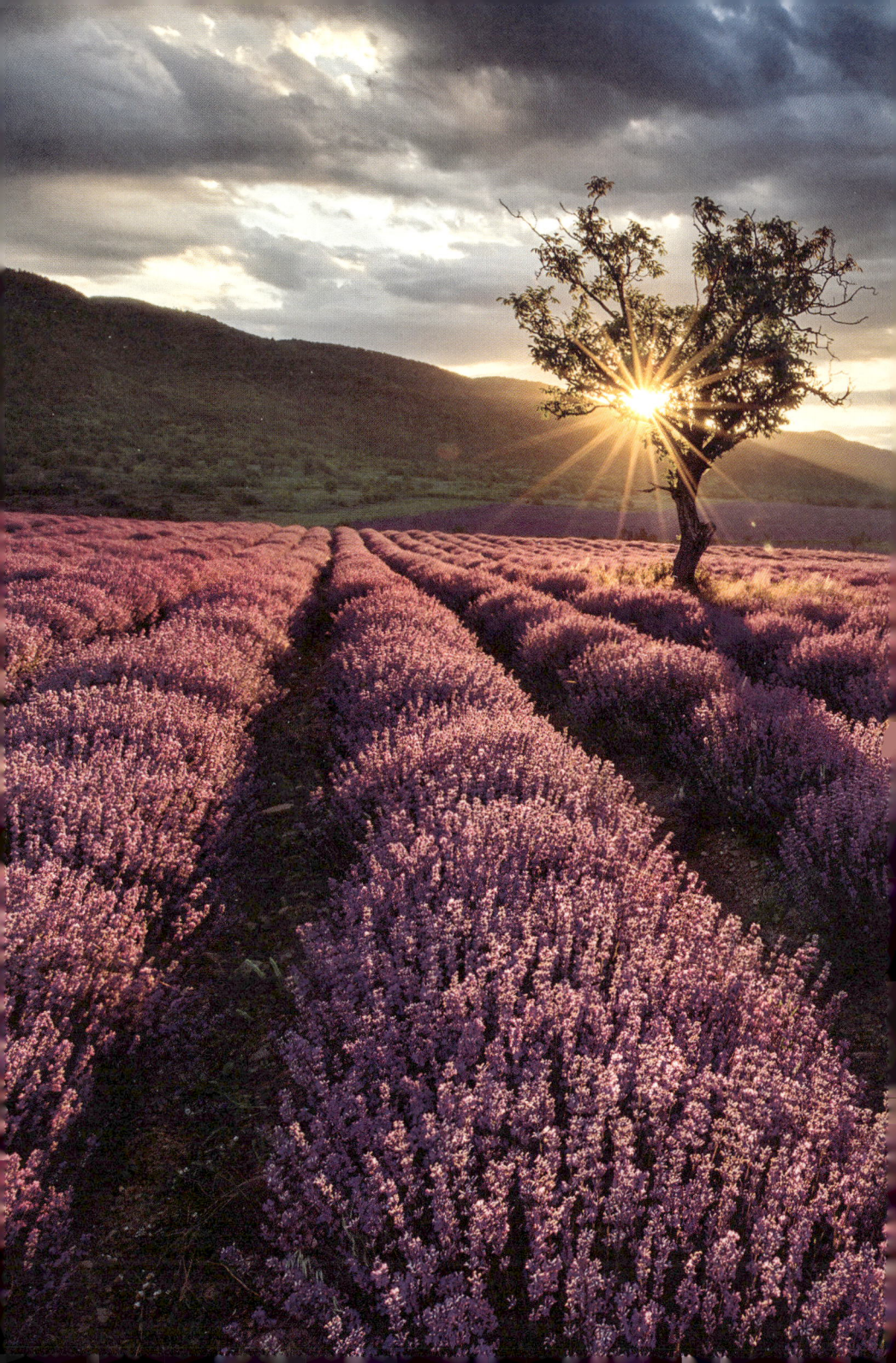

Chapter 3
Extraction of Essential Oils

Essential oils are called the "ruh" of the plant, meaning the soul. And rightfully so, as they carry its healing properties. Invisible to the naked eye, the volatile molecules of the plant precipitate in the form of essential oils captured through different methods used to extract oils from various parts of the plant. A classic example is the orange tree, which gives us three fabulous and unique oils. The peel of the orange fruit gives us Orange oil, the leaf from the same tree provides Petitgrain oil, and the flowers give us Neroli oil, commonly called Orange Blossom oil. All these oils are extracted using different methods from the same tree. Extracting the oils from their source is the first step in the process of bottling essential oils. Oil from each of these sources is extracted using a specific method.

1) Cold Press Method

The cold press method, one of the simplest oil extraction methods, is primarily used for citrus fruits. Its straightforward process provides reassurance about its ease of use.

Process:

As the name suggests, the process involves taking the peel of the fruit (orange, lemon, lime, grapefruit) and mechanically crushing it to extract the oil present in the small pouches, giving access to the pure oil. It is called cold press extraction, as no heat is involved. The only disadvantage of this method is that the oil extracted is highly volatile and has a short shelf life of only six to twelve months.

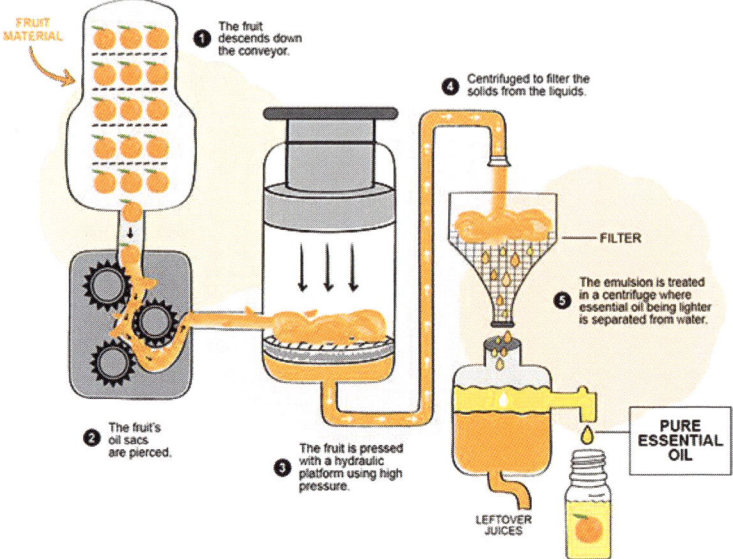

Image for representation of process only

2) Solvent Extraction

Solvent Extraction is a method mainly used for flowers where extracting their oils through any other method becomes complicated. This method is particularly useful for flowers with delicate structures.

Process:

Freshly plucked flowers are put into huge metal containers, and a highly deodorised solvent, such as hexane, is poured over them. The solvent extracts the wax from the flowers, which is then taken for vacuum processing, separating the solvent from the wax. The solvent is then reused. The remaining wax is called concrete, which contains a high percentage of essential oil. After this step, absolute alcohol separates oil from the wax, and you get oils called 'absolute'. To technically differentiate the extraction process, the word absolute is used after the name of the plant (generally flower) oil.

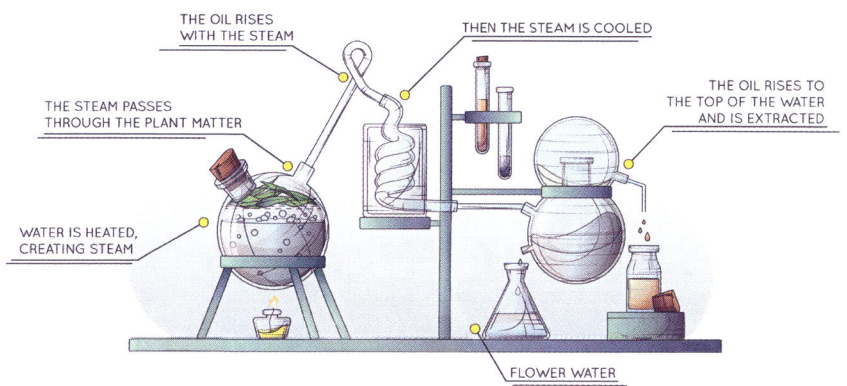

Image for representation of process only

3) Steam Distillation

Steam distillation is a cornerstone technique in aromatherapy. It preserves delicate aromatic compounds and ensures the purity and potency of the oils. It is widely used to extract oils from different parts of plants, such as leaves, roots, stems, berries, etc., to produce high-quality, therapeutic-grade essential oils.

Process:

Plant material is placed in a still, resting on a grid. Steam from boiling water is directed to the grid and passed through the raw material. Heat breaks down the essential oil and liberates most of its volatile, fragrant compounds. The condensate from distillation, which contains water and aromatic molecules, settles in a florence flask. This allows for easy separation of the fragrant oils from the water as, in most cases, the oil will float to the top of the distillate from where it is removed, leaving behind the water distillate. The water collected from the condensate, which retains some of the fragrant compounds and oils from the raw material, is called hydrosol and is sometimes sold for consumer and commercial use or is retrieved for reuse. However, a few essential oils (denser than water) will sink and be trapped at the bottom of a florentine vase. In all cases, the result is what we would term "a pure essential oil."

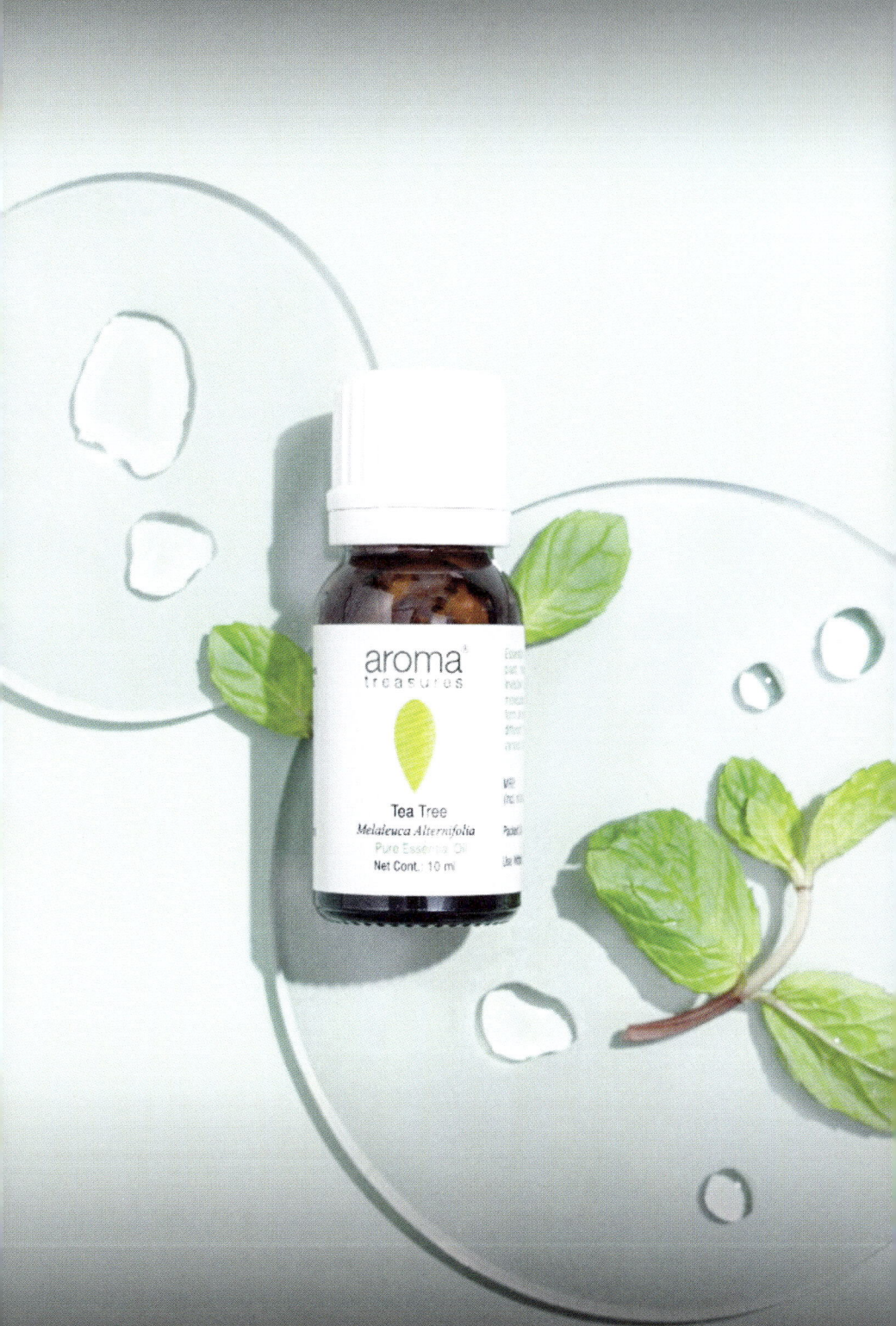

Chapter 4

Simple and Effective Methods of Using Essential Oils

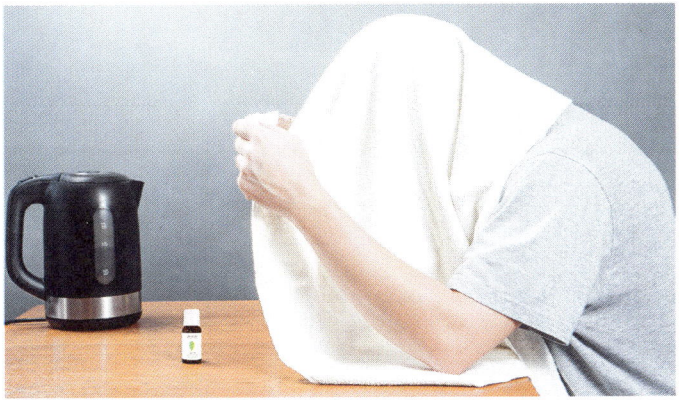

1. Vaporization

In a tea light, electric or steam diffuser, add four drops of either a single or a mixture of essential oils (without carrier oil) with a bit of water to diffuse the oil molecules in the room. Keep the door and windows closed to prevent the vapours from escaping. Within fifteen to twenty minutes, the oil will be diffused, and the healing properties of the oil shall prove themselves. This method also destroys bacteria and prevents the spread of infection in the air.

2. Steam Inhalation

Take some steaming water in a bowl or use a steamer, add three drops of essential oils (without carrier oil), and add to water. Cover your head with the towel, lean over the bowl or steamer, and inhale, keeping your eyes closed.

3. On Tissue

Put two drops of essential oil (without carrier oil) on the tissue and sniff regularly, or place it near your pillow before sleeping.

4. Bath

Bathing with essential oils is a beautiful experience. It is relaxing and can relieve aches, pain, balance emotions, and heal skin problems. People who do not have a bathtub should add three drops of oil in a teaspoon of vegetable oil. After washing the soap from the body, apply the mixture all over, or add five to six drops of the chosen essential oils to your bucket of water after washing soap from the body and let warm water run over you. Then, lightly dab your body so oils do not get wiped out. The best way is to add the oil mixture to a tub of warm water and stay in it for as long as you desire. The oil molecules are absorbed by the skin and through the lungs, which go directly into the bloodstream.

5. Body Massage

Essential oils stimulate skin cells to reproduce quicker, thus reducing the time lag between new skin growth and eliminating old cells. Skin treated with essential oils thus becomes more dynamic and strong. Essential oils can prevent the congestion of toxins and expedite the elimination of toxic debris by improving the lymphatic flow and general condition of the lymph glands. They neutralize unwanted unfriendly bacteria, prevent blemish conditions, and act as anti-inflammatories. They calm sensitive and damaged skin. They help relieve stress and tension that often lead to ageing skin. Collagen and elastin are kept in good condition, and there is some basis to believe that the nutrients and proteins contained in essential oils work as restorative building blocks to these important tissue fibres. After treatment with these oils, the body goes through a

Simple and Effective Methods of Using Essential Oils

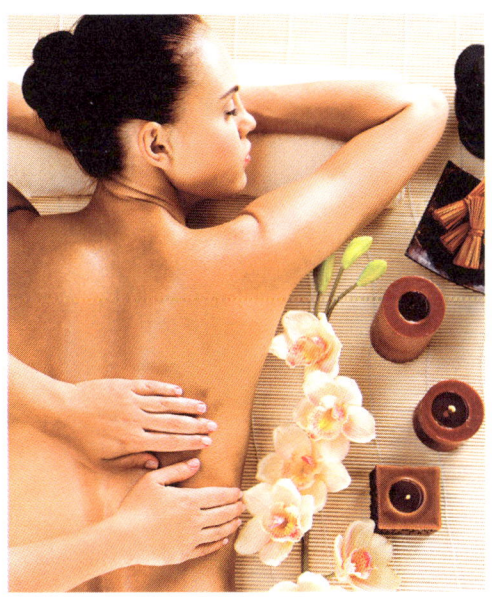

fundamental change, sometimes so dramatic that it seems the person has had a facelift.

Massage is helpful for relaxation, insomnia, stress, aches, pain and sluggish circulation. Additionally, it acts as a digestive tonic and passive exercise. It is not always necessary to have a whole-body massage. You can benefit from parts of the body being massaged. For example, the abdomen can be massaged for gas and colic, or the legs when tired and aching. A back massage at bedtime is extremely beneficial to comfort and relax you for a good night's sleep. Take one to two teaspoons of carrier oil or moisturising lotion, add four to eight drops of a single oil or a blend of the essential oils as per your choice, and massage your body. If you plan to massage regularly, you could prepare a blend of 50 ml base and add approximately twenty five to thirty drops of essential oils. Be sure to store it in a dark-coloured bottle away from heat and sunlight.

6. Hair Treatment

For a head massage, add three drops of essential oils to 5 ml of carrier oil. Part your hair and apply the oil to the scalp, not forgetting the ends. Leave the oil for at least thirty minutes before washing. Add two to three drops of the oils to your shampoo for a single wash.

7. Compress

An aromatic compress can help with headaches, sprains, and bruising. Add essential oils to two cups of warm water, dip in a folded flannel, squeeze out the excess liquid, and lay the flannel over the area you need to treat.

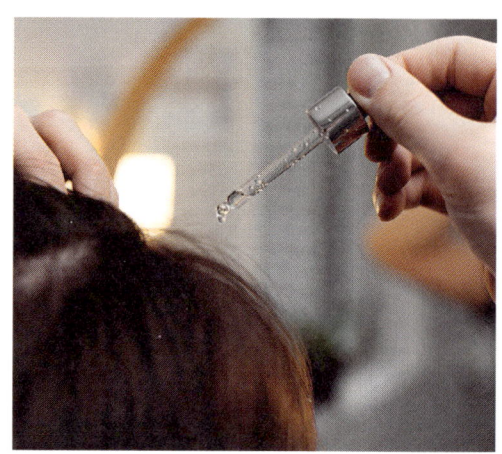

8. Skin Treatment

Essential oils can also be used in various ways to treat the skin. Skin cleansers help eliminate extra sweat and pollutants that are attracted to our face or cleansing toxins that accumulate on the face. Essential oils are widely incorporated into creams and lotions to imbue them with natural, therapeutic fragrances and leverage their potential skin benefits, such as moisturising, anti-inflammatory, and antibacterial properties. Facial scrubs are used to exfoliate the skin, unplug pores, and leave the skin looking fresh and dewy as the dead layer of cells is removed. It revitalizes the skin tone and helps rejuvenate the skin. Facial masks can nourish, rejuvenate, stimulate, refine, cleanse, and peel off the outer skin layer. They soothe inflamed skin, unclog blackheads, clear acne, and act as an anti-wrinkle treatment for a natural facelift. In all cases, a face mask improves the colour and tone of your face.

Simple and Effective Methods of Using Essential Oils

Safety and Precautions:

1. Essential oils are potent and should be used in low percentages. Before using on the skin, they should be diluted in a base oil/product.
2. Never use essential oils near or in the eyes, genital area, and other mucous membranes unless under the guidance of an aromatherapist.
3. Never use the oils internally. Keep out of reach of children.
4. Before using any oils, always check suitability for yourself and read any safety precautions/instructions regarding the oil.
5. Use as per the recommended dosages for adults, children, and those with sensitive skin.
6. Pure essential oils are needed for therapeutic effects, so buy only from a reputed supplier.
7. Essential oils should always be stored in dark glass bottles away from sunlight and other strong smells. The caps should be firmly in place to prevent evaporation.
8. Essential oils should not be used during the first twenty weeks of pregnancy. Even after twenty weeks, a professional aromatherapist should be consulted. Precautions and safety guidelines should be read properly before using essential oils.
9. A sprain should never be massaged. Always consult a doctor.
10. Some oils may irritate the skin. They must be used in a dilution of less than 1 per cent in a base oil or three drops maximum in a bath. These oils are unsuitable for highly sensitive skin and children–basil sweet, black pepper, cinnamon leaf, clove, eucalyptus, fennel, lemon, peppermint and pine.

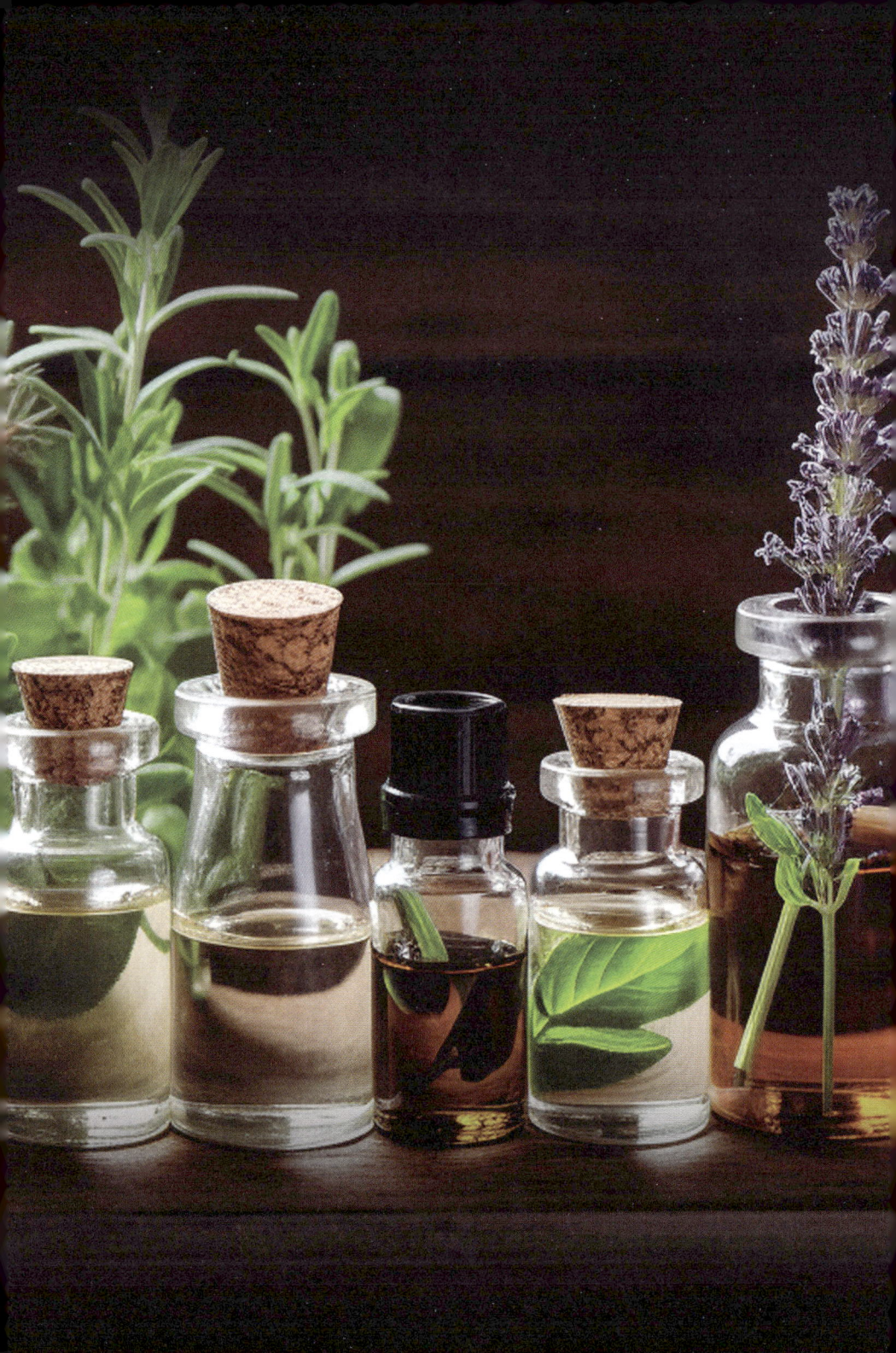

Chapter 5
Types of Essential Oils

Essential oils capture the essence of their source and offer myriad benefits for the mind, body, and spirit. These potent oils are categorized into various types based on their properties, uses and parts of the plant from which they are derived.

CITRUS

Derived from the peels of citrus fruits, these oils are refreshing and invigorating. Common citrus oils include lemon, orange, grapefruit, and bergamot. Citrus essential oils are widely used for their uplifting and mood enhancing effects and are often added to cleaning products, skincare items and diffusers.

Bergamot (Citrus Bergamia)

Family: Rutaceae | Perfumery note: top | Aroma: light citrus with a floral hint

The bergamot tree, with its ability to reach up to sixteen feet, shares close botanical ties with lemon and bitter orange trees. The process of extracting its essential oil involves the gentle expression, which is essentially squeezing of the rind from its green fruits, which resemble slightly oval-shaped oranges. Bergamot's name comes from the charming northern Italian town of Bergamot, where its precious oil was introduced to the market. The history of this aromatic citrus is intertwined with a more adventurous tale. Legend states that Christopher Columbus brought the first bergamot tree from the Canary Islands to Italy after one of his journeys.

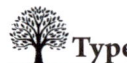

Since then, it has thrived in the sun-soaked regions of the country. In these southern parts of Italy, local communities initially employed bergamot for managing fevers, although its full range of healing properties was unveiled recently. Over time, it became a cherished ingredient in perfumery and played a vital role in the original formulation of Eau de Cologne. Furthermore, its delightful aroma contributes to the distinctive character of Earl Grey tea.

Main Qualities

Body/Skin

It is known to strengthen the immune system. Suitable for oily skin. Care must be taken when applying it to skin due to the risk of photosensitivity. Reduces colic. Beneficial for eczema and psoriasis due to stress.

Mind/Emotions

It combats fatigue caused by stress, tension, and anxiety. It brightens the mind and lifts the spirits, offering relief to those overwhelmed by problems. It's good for depression and brings good cheer, dispelling self-criticism and renewing a sense of happiness.

How To Use

Bath, compress, inhalation, massage, perfume, room fragrance, skincare preparations. It can cause photosensitivity, so be careful when applying it to the skin before exposure to sunlight.

Grapefruit (Citrus Paradisi)

Family: Rutaceae | Perfumery note: top | Aroma: citrus sharp, sweet

This impressive tree can reach heights of up to forty feet and has dark green, glossy, oval-shaped leaves with large yellow fruit.

The essential oil is extracted through cold expression, which involves squeezing the fruit's rind.

Grapefruit is believed to have originated from the pomelo *(Citrus grandis)*, originally native to Asia. The pomelo was larger than today's grapefruit and had sour yet refreshing flesh, which is popular in India. Captain Shaddock is credited with introducing the fruit to the West Indies, where it became known as 'shaddock fruit'. Spanish settlers brought its seeds to the United States in 1809, but commercial cultivation didn't begin until 1880. Its high Vitamin C content, known for its protective effect against infectious illnesses, was recognized early on. In the early 1900s, 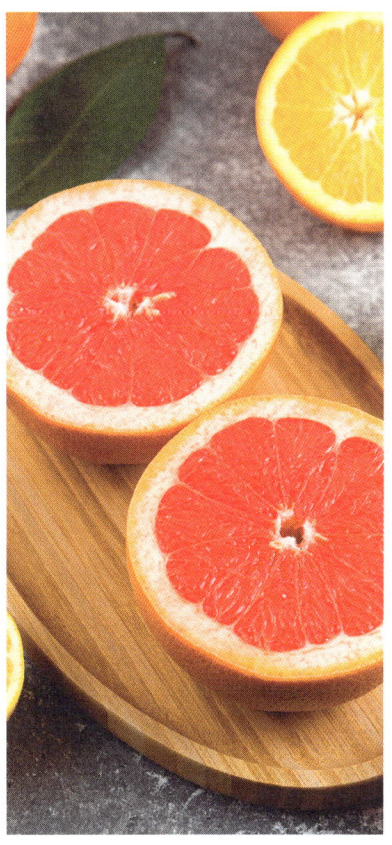 grapefruit gained popularity, leading to the canning of segments and juice production in Florida. Cultivation expanded to Texas, California, and Israel, where most grapefruit oil is produced today.

Main Qualities

Body/Skin

It helps treat oily skin and hair and is often recommended for cellulite blends because of its toning and astringent effects.

Mind/Emotions

Energising and uplifting oil. Helpful in treating eating disorders, both anorexia

Types of Essential Oils

and overeating, stemming from a lack of self-esteem. It creates a feeling of internal joy.

How To Use

Bath, compress, inhalation, massage, perfume, room fragrance, skincare preparations. It can cause photosensitivity, so be careful when applying it to the skin before exposure to sunlight.

Lemon (Citrus Limonum)

Family: Rutaceae | Perfumery note: top | Aroma: fresh, sharp

This robust tree can reach heights of up to sixteen feet, boasting the familiar fruit and beautifully scented flowers. Lemon essential oil is obtained through cold expression, squeezing the fruit's peel. Originally from Asia, lemon trees now thrive in the Mediterranean region and are extensively cultivated in Israel and the Americas. Lemon is closely related to bergamot and shares similar qualities. Lemons are widely believed to contribute to overall good health. Originating in Asia, ancient Egyptians used lemons to prevent food poisoning and epidemics. Crusaders brought lemons to Europe in the Middle Ages, quickly spreading to Greece, Italy, Sicily, Spain, and Portugal. English sailors valued their high Vitamin C content as a preventive measure against scurvy on long voyages. This remedy was so successful that until the early 20th century,

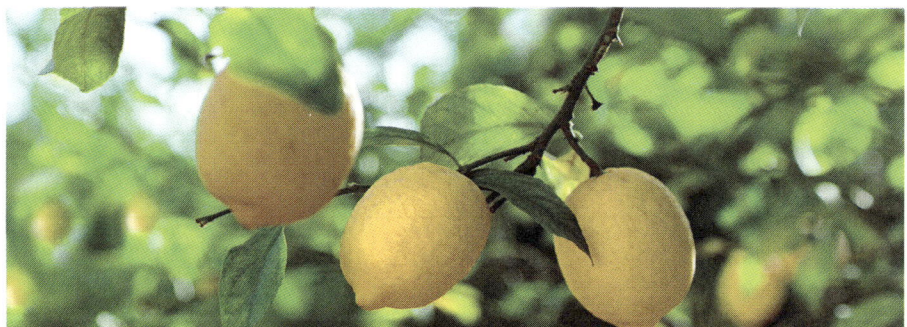

Types of Essential Oils

the British Navy mandated carrying enough lemon juice on ships for voyages lasting more than ten days. Externally, lemon has a mild skin-bleaching effect, making it helpful in whitening hands and fading freckles.

Main Qualities

Body/Skin

A good cleanser for skin and hair, especially in reducing dandruff. Beneficial for acne and oily skin.

Mind/Emotions

Brings clarity and stimulates the mind. Removes stress and depression. Refreshing and clarifying. Alleviates touchiness and feelings of resentment or bitterness about life's experiences.

How To Use

Bath, compress, hair care, insect repellent, massage, perfume, room fragrance, skincare, steam inhalation. It can cause photosensitivity, so be careful when applying it to the skin before exposure to sunlight.

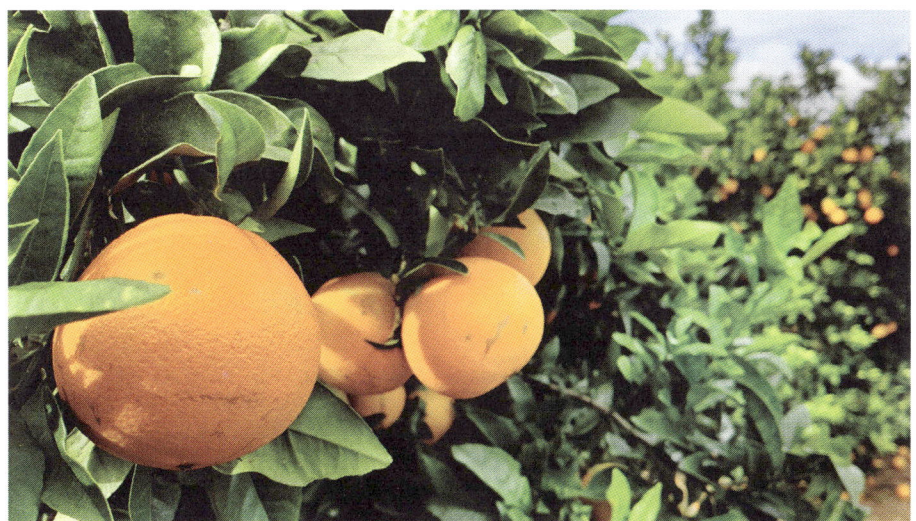

🍊 Orange (Citrus Sinensis)

Family: Rutaceae | Perfumery note: top | Aroma: refreshing, sweet, citrus

There are two types of orange trees: the sweet orange and the bitter orange. Essential oil is obtained from both of them through cold expression (literally squeezing).

The aroma described above is that of the sweet orange; the bitter variety has a more decadent, subtle scent. The latter also gives neroli oil from its fragrant blossoms and petitgrain oil from its leaves. Although native to China and the Middle East, these beautiful trees grow widely in Brazil, Mediterranean and USA. Over 4,000 years ago, Indians and Chinese used oranges for cosmetic and medicinal purposes. Columbus brought oranges to the West Indies, and by 1565, they were imported to Florida by the Spanish. Back in Europe, during plague outbreaks, the wealthy carried pomanders made from oranges stuck with cloves as protection from the disease. Queen Elizabeth I was said to wear one constantly, fixed to a long chain around her neck. In 1769, the tree was taken to the west of America and successfully cultivated by Franciscan monks; California and Florida are the world's significant producers today. The edible fruit containing high levels of vitamins comes from the sweet orange tree, whereas the bitter orange fruit is inedible. Both oils are used for perfumery, cosmetic manufacture and flavouring food.

Main Qualities

Body/Skin

Has relaxing properties and alleviates muscle and joint discomfort when applied as a massage oil.

Types of Essential Oils

Mind/Emotions

Used in an aroma lamp, it brightens the atmosphere of a room and is an antidepressant. Blended with spice or coniferous oils, it makes a wonderful holiday blend. Orange is refreshing and relaxing.

How To Use

Bath, compress, inhalation, massage, perfume, room fragrance, skincare preparations. It can cause photosensitivity, so be careful when applying it to the skin before exposure to sunlight.

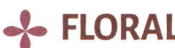 FLORAL

Extracted from flowers, these oils are known for their calming and soothing properties. Floral essential oils are often used in aromatherapy to reduce stress and promote relaxation, making them ideal to use in diffusers, bath products, and massage oils.

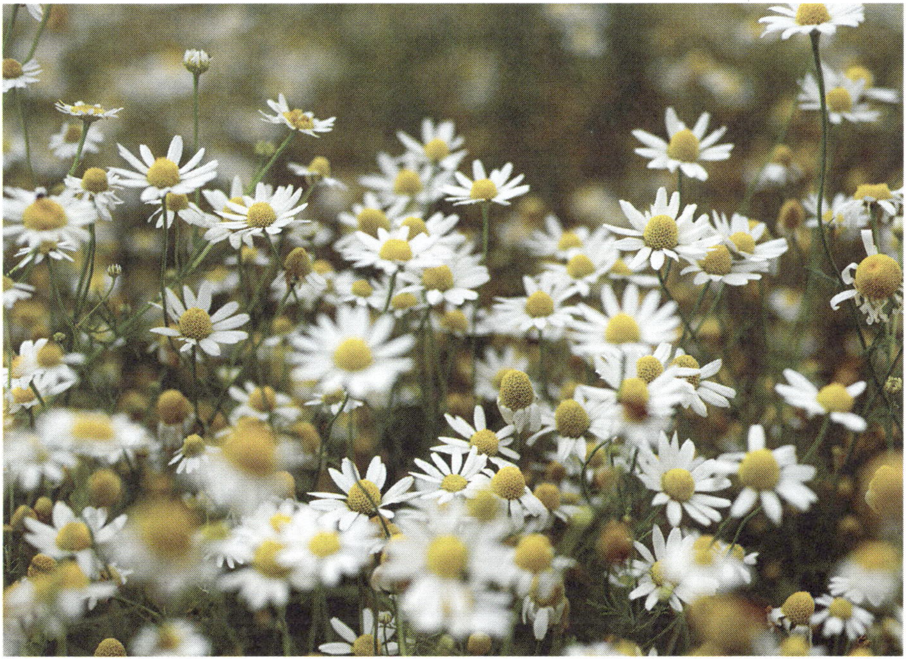

✣ Chamomile German (Matricaria Chamomille)

Family: Compositae | Perfumery note: middle | Aroma: musty, strong and herbaceous

Chamomile German, a cherished member of the daisy family, is derived from delicate flowers through steam distillation. What sets Chamomile German apart is its enchanting deep blue hue, a visual testament to its unique properties. Chamomile oil was commonly used until WWII as a natural disinfectant in hospitals and surgeries, as its antiseptic power was 120 times that of sea or salt water. It can also be used in potpourri and was listed as a clothes freshener in Edward III's household accounts.

Main Qualities
Body/Skin

The oil is excellent for treating inflamed, irritated skin. Dilute it in a carrier oil or use it in a compress for any inflammation. It excels at treating dry, itchy, and flaky skin problems and helps regenerate tissue. This oil is best when added to a blend for infected skin and acne. It can also be blended with lavender to treat sunburn.

Mind/Emotions

It has calming and sedating properties. When used in a diffuser along with lavender, it helps calm overexcited children.

How To Use

Bath, compress, hair care, massage, perfume, room fragrance, skincare.

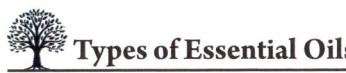

✦ Chamomile Roman (Anthemis Nobilis)

Family: Compositae | Perfumery note: middle | Aroma: fairly sweet with a hint of apple

The oil from Chamomile Roman gracefully transforms from blue into a soft yellow as it matures. Renowned for its remarkable versatility across the ages, chamomile stands as one of the most celebrated medicinal herbs. In ancient Greece, it bore the name 'apple of the Earth,' a poetic homage to its gentle and sweet fragrance. During the Middle Ages in England, chamomile found a place along pathways, allowing its soothing aroma to permeate the air with each footfall, a practice that benefits the plant's growth. Notably, even today, a chamomile lawn graces Buckingham Palace, a testament to the enduring allure of this botanical gem.

Main Qualities
Body/Skin

It is used for inhalation or as a sedative or pain reliever for intestinal spasms. It is helpful for inflammation and muscle and joint pains. It is useful to combat arthritis, menstrual cramps, and headaches. It is good for skin disorders, mainly dry and itchy skin. It soothes burns and acne.

Mind/Emotions

It is wonderful for insomnia caused by stress or tension. Roman is excellent for relaxing and summoning sleep.

How To Use

Bath, compress, hair care, massage, perfume, room fragrance, skincare.

✣ Jasmine Absolute (Jasminum Grandiflorum)

Family: Oleaceae | Perfumery note: middle | Aroma: rich, heady, and floral

A climbing shrub, jasmine can reach heights of approximately fifty two feet, with the oil derived from its small, white flowers. Jasmine has several varieties worldwide, but the oils from *Jasminum officinale* and *Jasminum grandiflorum* are favoured in aromatherapy. Jasmine is called the king of flowers. It is essential for anyone interested in perfumery but offers much more than a lovely exotic aroma. Jasmine flowers are harvested before dawn, when the oil yield is at its peak, requiring thousands of flowers to produce even a tiny amount of essential oil. A high-quality jasmine oil should have a deep orange-brown colour and a relatively thick consistency. Major producers include North Africa, Italy, India, Turkey, and China, but French oil is often considered superior. For centuries, the exquisite fragrance of jasmine has been renowned for its aphrodisiac qualities. As a result, jasmine flowers and oil have been prominent ingredients in love potions and sensual perfumes. Women in India also traditionally placed jasmine blossoms in their well-oiled hair to enhance their scent and display the beauty of the flowers. Jasmine holds sacred significance for devotees of Vishnu, who use the flowers as votive offerings in religious ceremonies. Intensely fragrant white jasmine flowers have been used in tea for centuries, their origins tracing back to ancient China during the Song Dynasty (960-1279 AD). Layering with tea leaves to naturally infuse the fragrance led to a luxurious blend favoured by Chinese nobility for its calming effects and exquisite aroma.

Main Qualities
Body/Skin

It is used in skincare, especially in treating dry skin. However, it can be sensitizing and is not recommended to use on problem skin.

Mind/Emotions

Some also recommend it as a "hormone balancer" that soothes menstrual pain. It is an excellent aphrodisiac, especially for those who lack confidence in their sexuality. It is also a powerful antidepressant, helps diminish fear and builds self-confidence and optimism.

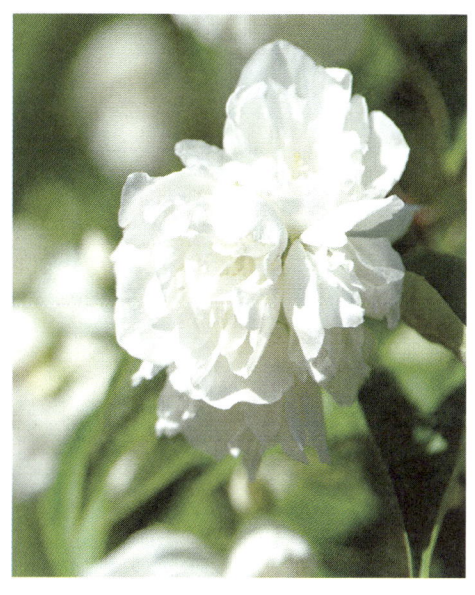

How To Use
Bath, compress, skincare, hair care, massage, perfume, room fragrance.

✣ Lavender (Lavandula Angustifolia)

Family: Iabiatae | Perfumery note: top/middle | Aroma: fresh, floral, sweet with herbaceous undertones

Several varieties of lavender are cultivated globally, but *Lavandula angustifolia*, also known as "true" lavender or Lavandulavera, or *Lavandula officinale*, is the preferred choice for aromatherapy. This type of lavender thrives at altitudes of around 3,000 feet and boasts beautiful lavender-coloured flowering tops. The essential oil is obtained through steam distillation of these flower tops.

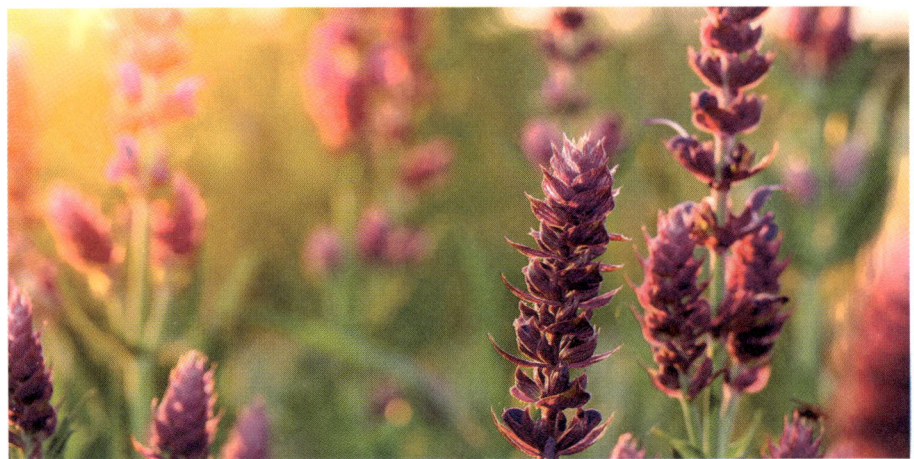

Lavender has enjoyed centuries of use owing to its remarkable versatility. Egyptians cultivated lavender in their walled gardens, using dried flowers for body oils and to perfume clothes. The Romans embraced lavender for bathing, coining the name from "lavare", meaning "to wash", but it was a luxury only the wealthiest women could afford. It was also used as an antidote for snake venom. In 14th century Europe, lavender's popularity grew further. Lavender featured prominently in cosmetics like Hungary Water, which was known for preserving the irresistible beauty of Queen Elizabeth of Hungary into her seventies. Queen Elizabeth I of England drank lavender tea for migraines, and it later became a favourite of Napoleon and Empress Josephine when incorporated into eau de cologne. While lavender water remains popular today, it reached the peak of fashion in the late 19th century. The remarkable healing properties of lavender oil were rediscovered almost by accident in the early 20th century by a French chemist named Gatefossé. He experienced rapid healing without scarring after accidentally immersing his burned arms in lavender oil following a laboratory explosion!

Main Qualities
Body/Skin

It is used on burns, minor abrasions, and skin problems. It is an essential component for acne treatment and an excellent addition to all types of skincare products. It is antibacterial, antifungal, and possibly antiviral. It soothes tired muscles and boosts the immune system.

Mind/Emotions

Used in bath oil, it is excellent for relaxing in the tub and for good sleep. Awakens harmony. It aids in restoring balance and calms the mind and body.

How To Use

Bath, compress, skincare, hair care, inhalation, massage, perfume, room fragrance.

✦ Mogra Absolute (Jasminum Sambac)

Family: Oleaceae | Perfumery note: middle | Aroma: floral, sweet, warm, exotic

A bit harsher than *Jasminum grandiflorum*, Mogra is a species of jasmine native to South Asia, Southeast Asia, and the Arabian Peninsula. Mogra essential oil is extracted by solvent extraction due to the delicate nature of the flower. It holds a special place in the aromatherapy and perfumery worlds due to its rich, sweet, captivating scent and deep floral notes. "Jasmine" originates from the Arabic "Yasmin", translating to "Gift from God". In India, *Jasmine sambac*, mogra, is revered as the "Queen of the Night" for its intensified fragrance after sunset. In the Philippines, known as Sampaguita, or "I promise you", the flower epitomizes loyalty, purity, and undying love. In Chinese culture, jasmine represents the sweetness of women, while in India, it signifies divine hope. By the 15th century, jasmine was a coveted addition to the imperial gardens of China, Iran, Afghanistan and Nepal, celebrated for its aromatic blossoms.

**Main Qualities
Mind/Emotions**

It is good for stress and depression. It boosts confidence and brings joy and happiness. It is an excellent aphrodisiac.

How To Use

Bath, compress, skincare, hair care, massage, perfume, room fragrance.

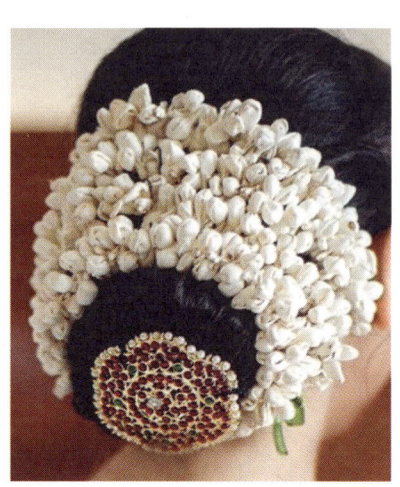

✣ Neroli (Citrus Aurantium)

Family: Rutaceae | Perfumery note: middle | Aroma: floral, bittersweet, a beautiful (non-citrus) scent

Bitter orange, scientifically known as *Citrus vulgaris* or *bigaradia* is also referred to as Seville orange. Neroli, or orange blossom oil, is extracted from this tree's fragrant, white flowers. Originally native to China, it now thrives throughout the Mediterranean region. Notably, it takes approximately one tonne of hand-picked blossoms to produce just one kg of oil. The name originates from Anne-Marie Orsini, the Duchess of Nerola in Italy. She was of French descent and had an immense fondness for the scent of orange blossoms. Her affection for this fragrance led her to scent her bathwater, gloves, and clothing with orange blossoms. This practice quickly caught on among the aristocracy, making the orange blossom scent highly fashionable and sought after. It worked as a good toner. However, the allure of neroli was recognized long before this time. Legend has it that Cleopatra frequently used a heady and exotic body oil made from orange blossoms, honey, and cinnamon. Throughout centuries, it became customary in Europe for brides to wear or carry orange blossoms as symbols of purity and loveliness.

The scent of these blossoms was believed to calm nerves and bring joy to newlyweds on their wedding night. Even Napoleon, the Emperor of France, had a strong affection for the scent of violets and neroli in his favourite cologne, which he liberally used even during military campaigns. Neroli, often blended with bergamot, lavender, and rosemary, was also a key component in the original Eau de Cologne.

Main Qualities
Body/Skin

Neroli has a sebum-balancing effect, which can help balance oily and dry skin. It is also beneficial for dry sensitive skin and stretch marks.

Mind/Emotions

Can help calm anxiety and relieve depression. Key ingredient in antianxiety blends. Helps induce sleep for insomniacs, acting as a natural tranquilliser.

How To Use

Bath, compress, skincare, hair care, massage, perfume, room fragrance.

✣ Rose Absolute (Rosa Damascena)

Family: Rosaceae | Perfumery note: middle | Aroma: rich, floral, sweet, an exquisite scent

There are hundreds of rose varieties worldwide, but two fragrant types are commonly used in aromatherapy: damask rose *(Rosa damascena),* also known as Bulgarian or Turkish rose, and cabbage rose *(Rosa centifolia),* sometimes referred to as Rose Maroc or Rose de Mai. These roses are typically harvested before dawn when the flowers are oil rich. It can take approximately one tonne of petals to produce just 500 gms of oil. Essences are obtained from the petals of both of these shrubs through steam distillation or a method using volatile solvents like liquid carbon dioxide.

Types of Essential Oils

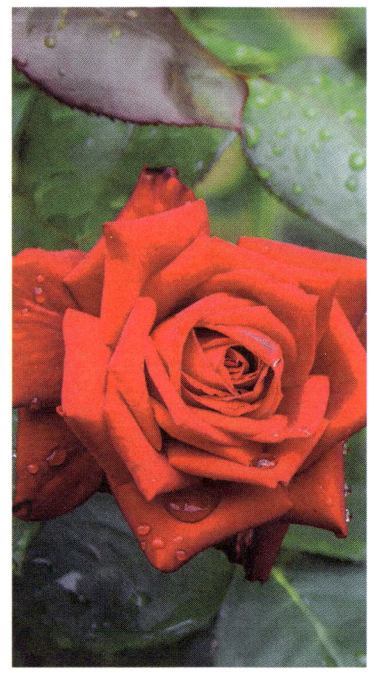

The former produces an oil known as an "otto", and the latter as an "absolute". Understanding this distinction is useful when purchasing rose oil. Bulgarian rose "otto" is often considered the finest in the world and is therapeutically superior to the fragrant rose, Maroc absolute. Rosewater is also produced for the cosmetic and food industries, with the best-quality rosewater from France. Rose oil is primarily produced in Morocco, Bulgaria, Egypt, China, India, France, and Russia. The rose, often called the "queen of flowers", has a rich history and has been associated with beauty and love for centuries.

In ancient Egypt, rose body oils were used, and Cleopatra, the famous Egyptian queen, is said to have covered her bedroom floor with rose petals before seducing Julius Caesar. In ancient Rome, roses were added to wine, clothes were soaked in rosewater for fragrance, and rose petals were scattered on marriage beds. Roses were also used to sweeten the breath, and Arab healers believed rose jam could heal lung complaints. The rose was introduced to Europe during the Crusades, where it was used medicinally in decoctions for various ailments. Throughout history, roses have been a symbol of beauty and love in art and literature, with poets and playwrights extolling their virtues. Roses continue to be cherished for their beauty, fragrance, and symbolism in various cultures and are used in a wide range of products, including perfumes, cosmetics, and aromatherapy oils.

Main Qualities
Body/Skin

In Europe, it is used to treat genito-urinary infections. Sexual difficulties also respond well to rose oil's gentle support. It is good for dry skin, especially for delaying wrinkles.

Mind/Emotions

The ultimate woman's oil: calming and supportive and has no parallel in treating grief, hysteria or depression. It helps balance female hormones, regulates the menstrual cycle, and eases the discomforts of PMS and menopause.

How To Use

Bath, compress, skincare, hair care, massage, perfume, room fragrance.

✤ Tuberose (Polianthes Tuberosa)

Family: Asparagaceae | Perfumery note: middle | Aroma: sweet, floral, heady

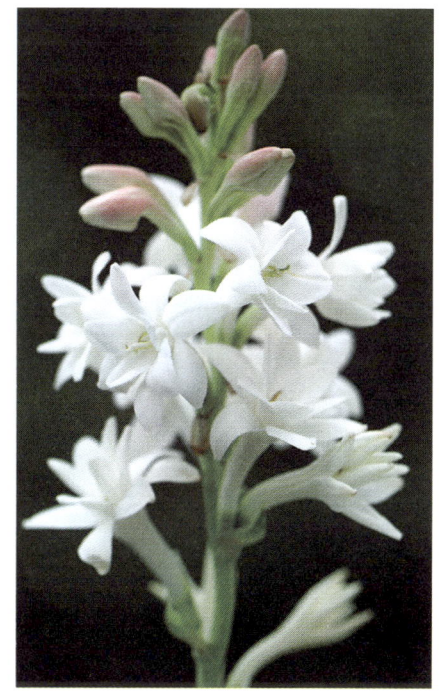

Tuberose is a perennial plant cherished for its fragrant, showy white flowers. Native to Mexico, tuberose has found a revered place in gardens and perfumeries worldwide, thriving in warm climates. The plant grows from bulbs, producing tall, slender stems crowned with creamy white, waxy flower clusters. From late summer into fall, tuberose flowers unfurl at dusk, releasing an intoxicating, heady scent that fills the night air.

Its potent, sweet aroma has made it a staple in the perfume industry, where it is valued for its depth and lasting power. Tuberose essential oil, extracted through enfleurage or solvent extraction due to the delicate nature of the flowers, is a luxurious ingredient in many high-end fragrances, lending them a sensual character. In addition to its olfactory appeal, tuberose has cultural and symbolic significance in various parts of the world. In India, for example, it is often used in wedding ceremonies and religious offerings; symbolising purity, sensuality, and fertility. In Mexico, tuberose is a popular adornment in religious and festive occasions, embodying joy and celebration. It has also been used in traditional medicine in some cultures and is believed to possess healing properties that help relax the mind, ease tension, and promote restful sleep.

Main Qualities
Body/Skin

Effective in treating impotence or frigidity.

Mind/Emotions

Works as an aphrodisiac;

Its sensual aroma can be a beautiful addition to blends for relaxation and romance. Promotes assertiveness, confidence, self-esteem.

How To Use

Bath, compress, hair care, massage, perfume, room fragrance, skincare.

✤ Ylang Ylang (Cananga Odorata)

Family: Annonaceae | Perfumery note: middle | Aroma: rich, sweet and floral, similar to jasmine

The ylang ylang tree *(Cananga odorata)* is known for its tall stature (sixty feet) and highly fragrant yellow flowers. Ylang Ylang essential oil is obtained through the steam distillation of its blossoms. While native to Asia, particularly the

Types of Essential Oils

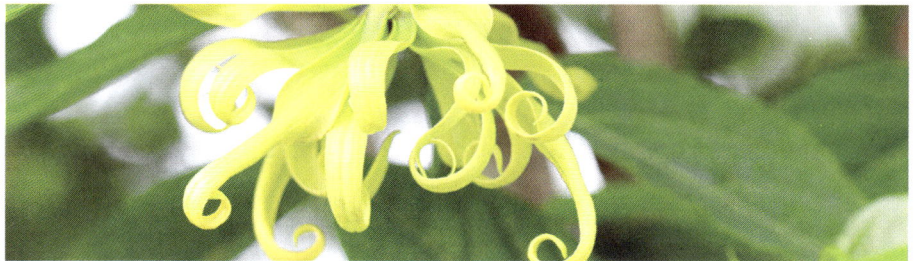

Philippines, ylang ylang oil is also produced in other tropical regions, including the Comoro Islands and Réunion in the Indian Ocean. This essential oil is valued for its exotic and sweet floral scent and is used in perfumery and aromatherapy. Ylang Ylang, also known as the "flower of flowers" or the "perfume tree", is renowned for its fragrant and drooping blossoms. Traditionaly, the women of Tahiti have used ylang ylang essential oil for hair care, often blending it with sandalwood and coconut oils to condition and scent their hair. Ylang Ylang is a prized ingredient in high-quality perfumes used to fragrance toiletries.

Main Qualities
Body/Skin

It lowers blood pressure and eases muscle spasms and tense muscles. It also treats PMS and menopausal symptoms. In facial oil or cream, it helps balance sebum production and is helpful for oily skin. It can fight bacteria that contribute to acne and stimulate hair growth. However, it should be avoided on sensitive skin.

Mind/Emotions

Antidepressant, relaxing to body, mind and spirit, as well as an aphrodisiac. Calms anger, releases tension, alleviates depression and stabilizes mood swings. Acts on the emotional heart centre, healing feelings of guilt, jealousy, resentment, and selfishness. Ylang ylang mixed with jasmine or rose has been used to treat sexual difficulties, especially those stemming from a lack of confidence.

How To Use

Bath, compress, skincare, hair care, massage, perfume, room fragrance.

🌿 HERBACEOUS

These oils are obtained from the leaves, grass, twigs, berries or stems of plants/trees. Herbaceous essential oils are known for their stimulating and clarifying properties, often used to improve focus and mental clarity in diffusers, massage blends and topical applications.

🌿 Basil Sweet (Ocimum Basilicum)

Family: Labiatae | Perfumery note: middle | Aroma: clear, herbal

Among the many varieties of basil, some stand out for their aromatic qualities, with one in particular highly prized in aromatherapy, true sweet basil. The essential oil from sweet basil is obtained through meticulous steam distillation, focusing on the herbs delicate flowering tops and leaves. Basil derives its name from the Latin word "basilisca", meaning "royal". The ancient Greeks considered basil the antidote to the venom of the mythical Basilisk, a deadly reptile feared for its lethal breath and gaze.

Main Qualities
Body/Skin

Used in moderation, it helps ease sinus congestion and headaches. It is helpful against colds as well as easing muscular aches and pains. It helps in reducing menstrual cramps. Avoid usage if pregnant or subject to seizures.

Mind/Emotions

Basil is helpful for mental and physical fatigue, aiding mental alertness and concentration. It's an excellent wake-up oil, clearing the muddled mind. Encourages positivity, assertiveness, trust, integrity, enthusiasm.

How To Use

Bath, compress, skincare, massage, perfume, room fragrance.

Basil (Tulsi) (Ocimum Sanctum)

Family: Labiatae | Perfumery note: middle | Aroma: clear, herbal

The bushy, aromatic basil herb grows to about eighteen inches in height and flourishes in warm, tropical climates. It is easily identifiable by its vibrant green, oval-shaped leaves and delicate purple or white flowers. The essential oil is obtained through steam distillation of the leaves and flowering tops of the plant and has a distinctive earthy and sweet aroma with hints of mint and clove. Tulsi plays a significant role in magical and religious ceremonies. In Hindu culture, it is believed to offer protection from malevolent spirits. Basil plants were grown in households, and daily offerings of flowers were made to honour this sacred herb. This essential oil retains the therapeutic qualities of Tulsi, making it highly valued in aromatherapy, skincare, and holistic medicine. It alleviates stress, boosts immunity, and improves respiratory health. This sacred herb embodies the fusion of cultural heritage and natural healing, a testament to the rich botanical knowledge of India. In Hinduism, Tulsi is the manifestation of the Goddess Lakshmi. According to the Shrimad Devi Bhagavatam, a curse transformed Goddess Lakshmi into a tulsi plant. In another version of the legend, Vrinda immolates herself in her husband's funeral pyre, and Vishnu ensures she is reincarnated as a tulsi plant.

Main Qualities
Body/Skin

It also promotes the removal of catarrh matter and phlegm from bronchial tubes.

Mind/Emotions

It is a nerve tonic and is used to sharpen memory.

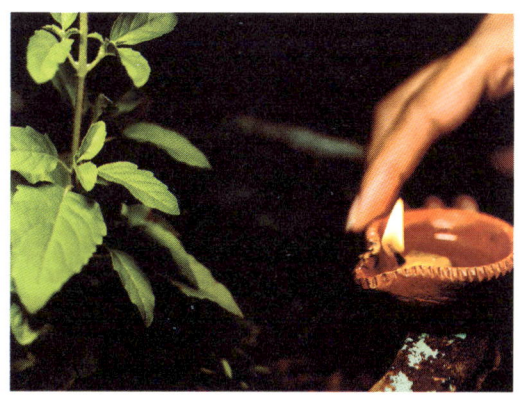

How To Use

Bath, compress, hair care, massage, perfume, room fragrance, skincare.

🌿 Carrot Seed (Daucus Carota)

Family: Umbelliferae | Perfumery note: middle | Aroma: earthy, warm, spicy

Carrot seed oil is extracted using steam distillation from the dried seeds of the wild carrot. This plant, which can grow to a height of three feet, boasts small white and deep purple flowers. Carrots are celebrated for their rich nutritional and medicinal benefits. Their journey began in Afghanistan, eventually gaining recognition in ancient Greece and Rome. The wild carrot, distinguishable by its small, hard, elongated white roots and intense aroma, can still be found across Europe, particularly in chalky soils near coastlines. The Dutch cultivated the modern orange carrot with its familiar tubular shape, crisp flesh, sweet aroma, and taste in the 17th century. White, deep purple, and red varieties are also grown in Europe. The wildflower known as Queen Anne's lace, prevalent along New World roadsides, is the wild carrot introduced by English colonists. Carrots are hardy biennials and among the simplest vegetables to cultivate at home. In 16th century France, carrots were revered as a nervous system tonic. Their reputed benefits for eyesight became legendary during World War II, with pilots reportedly consuming carrots to enhance their night vision.

Main Qualities

Body/Skin

Carrot seed oil is the best essential oil for caring for mature skin. It is excellent in dry skin blends. It is believed to stimulate the red blood cells, adding tone and elasticity to the skin. It reduces and prevents wrinkles. It is known for its regenerative powers after severe burns. Very good for removing scars. It also benefits dry hair and dandruff.

Types of Essential Oils

How To Use

Bath, compress, hair care, massage, perfume, room fragrance, skincare.

🌱 Citronella (Cymbopogon Nardus)

Family: Poaceae | Perfumery note: middle | Aroma: grassy, lemony, crispy

Citronella, a member of the family of aromatic and oil-rich tropical grasses, comes in several varieties. Typically robust and coarse, these plants can reach heights of four to five feet. They thrive in wild highland areas but are predominantly cultivated near coastal regions. Propagation is achieved through root division, and the grass is usually ready for harvest approximately eight months after planting, with subsequent harvests every four months, depending on the weather. These plants generally require replanting every four to five years. The most highly regarded varieties of citronella are found in Java, Sri Lanka, the Seychelles, New Guinea, and Guyana. In 1933, around 30,000 acres in Sri Lanka were dedicated to citronella cultivation. By 1987, exports of citronella oil reached between 100 and 120 tonnes. However, since then, both cultivation and production have seen a decline. Distilled from the grass, the oil ranges from yellow to dark brown and has a potent, aromatic, lemony fragrance. Its oil production can vary from season to season. Citronella oil is known for its strong, lemon-like scent that is effective in repelling mosquitoes while being pleasantly aromatic to humans.

Main Qualities
Body/Skin

Insect repellent

Mind/Emotions

Refreshes the mind. Induces feelings of freshness, happiness, and hope.

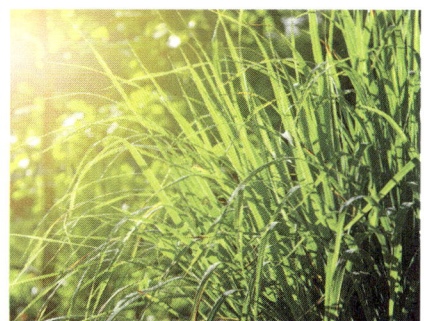

How To Use

Bath, compress, hair care, massage, perfume, room fragrance, skincare.

Clary Sage (Salvia Sclarea)

Family: Labiateae | Perfumery note: middle/base | Aroma: light, spicy, like drying hay

Clary Sage essential oil is obtained through steam distillation of the lilac flowering tops and leaves of a biennial herb with large wrinkled leaves, growing in England, Europe, Russia and USA. It is related to, but different from, the common sage used in cooking. The name "clary" likely originates from the Latin word "clarus," meaning "clear". The seeds were once used in a remedy to clear particles from the eyes. Introduced to Britain in 1562, this herb gained popularity for its remarkable ability to clear foreign bodies from the eyes, earning it the nickname "clear eye". Interestingly, in Germany, some merchants added clary and elder flowers to their wine to mimic the taste of the more expensive muscatel wine. However, this concoction led to dangerous levels of intoxication and severe hangovers. Consequently, clary sage is still referred to as "Muskateller Salbei" or "muscatel sage" in Germany. A similar wine known as "clary", crafted from ingredients like clary sage, honey, ginger, and pepper, gained popularity in 16th century England.

Main Qualities
Body/Skin

Essential for every woman, it helps ease menstrual cramps, balance PMS, and reduce the pangs of menopause. It has hormonal properties that can help balance menstrual and menopausal difficulties. It helps with dry and mature skin. It also benefits dry hair and dandruff.

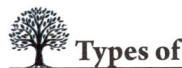

Mind/Emotions

Added to Geranium to balance extreme emotions, reduce stress and restore inner tranquillity. It helps clear confusion and false beliefs, guiding you towards new paths and potentials, and is used to combat depression. Particularly indicated for times of change, occupational and biological, and when having difficulty in adjusting to changes in life. *Warning: Avoid usage while consuming alcohol, and avoid use while pregnant.*

How To Use

Bath, compress, skincare, hair care, massage, perfume, room fragrance.

Cypress (Cupressus Sempervirens)

Family: Cupressaceae | Perfumery note: middle | Aroma: clear, yet woody with a hint of spice

Cypress, an evergreen tree that can reach heights of up to fifty eight feet, yields its essential oil by distilling its needles and twigs. Mediterranean countries abound with these striking trees, commonly associated with cemeteries and funerals as mourning symbols and traditionally believed to have supplied the wood for Christ's cross. Historical records trace the use of cypress to 4,000 years ago when the Babylonians imported it. In Roman and Greek cultures, the cypress was linked to death and the afterlife, possibly representing death as a transformative process.Its Latin name, "ever living", reflects its perpetual greenery throughout the year. Cypress's medicinal properties have a rich history. Hippocrates endorsed its use for healing uterine problems and haemorrhoids, while centuries later, Culpeper noted its effectiveness in preventing gum bleeding and securing loose teeth.

Main Qualities
Body/Skin

A known astringent, excellent for oily skin and useful for circulatory and respiratory problems. It is often used in blends to ease arthritis pain. It can ease the pain of aching muscles or menstrual cramps.

Mind/Emotions

It is comforting in times of loss and grief, helping you let go and process bottled-up emotions, encouraging you to trust the ebb and flow of life. It is excellent for increasing concentration and alleviating fear of what others think.

How To Use

Bath, compress, inhalation, massage, insect repellent, perfume, room fragrance, skincare.

Eucalyptus (Eucalyptus Globulous)

Family: Myrtceae | Perfumery note: top | Aroma: clearing, sharp, like camphor

Towering up to 380 feet, eucalyptus yields its essence through steam distillation of its oil-rich leaves and twigs. While there are over thirty eucalyptus varieties globally, only a select few find use in aromatherapy. *Eucalyptus globulus*, *Eucalyptus dives,* and *Eucalyptus radiata* are becoming more popular. *Eucalyptus*

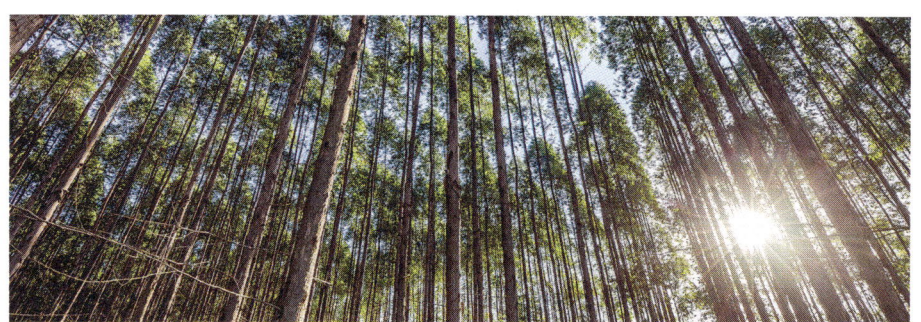

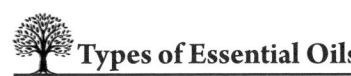
Types of Essential Oils

radiata, in particular, is valued in perfumery for its fresh, lemony scent. Eucalyptus, native to Australia and abundant in its forests, has been successfully introduced to other regions such as Africa, the Mediterranean and China. It was strategically planted in marshy areas plagued by malaria and infectious diseases, with remarkable results. The tree's roots absorbed excess water from the soil, while the leaves well-known scent transformed once "bug-stricken" areas into healthy oases. Eucalyptus is also called a gum tree because the bark exudes a sweet smelling gum. Aboriginal communities used eucalyptus leaves to bind around serious wounds for cleansing, infection prevention, and promoting swift healing. Pharmaceutical companies have long harnessed the potent healing properties of eucalyptus, incorporating them into many modern medicines and ointments in use today. The first works on the antiseptic and antibacterial properties of the oil were published in Germany by doctors Cloez (1870), Faust and Homeyer (1874).

Main Qualities
Body/Skin

Eucalyptus is best known for its respiratory effects. It fights viruses and bacteria while easing congestion. It also relieves muscle and joint aches and pains. Eucalyptus stimulates circulation, increasing the flow of blood to affected areas. It is also an excellent insect repellent.

Mind/Emotions

Eucalyptus can be mentally stimulating and may help increase concentration. *Warning: Do not use it with infants and small children; it can cause choking.*

How To Use

Bath, compress, insect repellent, massage, room fragrance, steam inhalation.

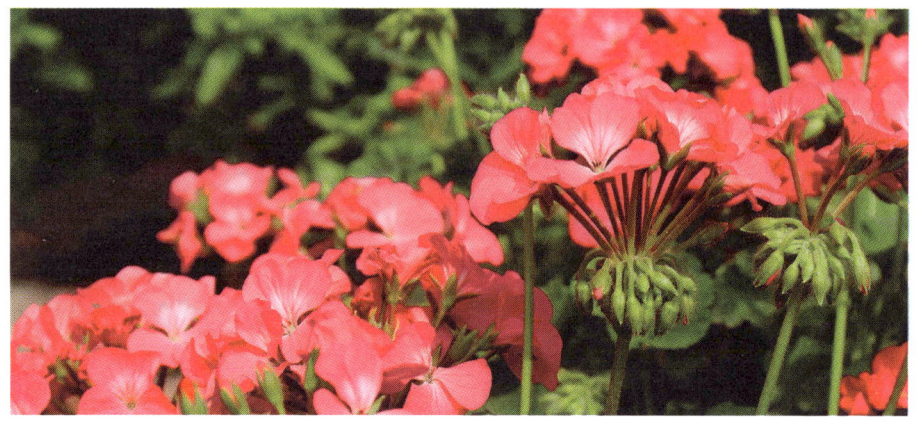

Geranium (Pelargonium Graveolens)

Family: Geraniaceae | Perfumery note: middle | Aroma: delicate floral, sweet and rose-like

Geranium is a herbaceous plant with pink flowers. The oil is distilled from the flowers, leaves and stalks of this attractive plant. Originally hailing from the Cape area of Africa, geraniums (more accurately called pelargoniums) were introduced to Europe in the 17th century, quickly gaining popularity.

Geranium oil is sometimes called "geranium bourbon" due to its historical cultivation on Île de Bourbon, now Reunion Island. The oil is still produced there and is known for its exceptional quality in perfumery. France, Morocco, Egypt and China are major exporters of geranium oil.

Main Qualities
Body/Skin

It is used for acne, burns and congestion. It is good for all kinds of skin and improves complexion. It acts as a diuretic. It lowers blood sugar and should be avoided if you are hypoglycemic.

Types of Essential Oils

Mind/Emotions

Balances physical and emotional conditions. It is an antidepressant and helps process feelings of fear and abandonment. It helps relieve fright, stress, induces sleep, and lowers blood pressure. It has a hormonal balancing effect and has traditionally been used (blended with clary sage) to alleviate problems associated with menopause and menstruation.

How To Use

Bath, compress, hair care, insect repellent, massage, perfume, room fragrance, skincare.

Juniper Berry (Juniperus Communis)

Family: Cupressaceae | Perfumery note: middle | Aroma: refreshing, crisp

This tree typically stands at heights ranging from six to fifteen feet, featuring delicate needle-like leaves and producing small berries. While the berries are green in the first year, they turn blue-black in successive years. Juniper berry oil is obtained through steam distillation of the berries, while juniper oil is extracted from the needle-like leaves and twigs. The essential oil derived from the berries is considered superior in therapeutic quality compared to the leaves and twigs. The ancient Egyptians employed juniper in combination with frankincense as a headache remedy. Juniper was also used in hair dye, a significant aspect of Egyptian physical appearance. In Tibet, juniper berries served as fabric dye. Many nations traditionally harnessed juniper, including temple incense, for medicinal and cleansing

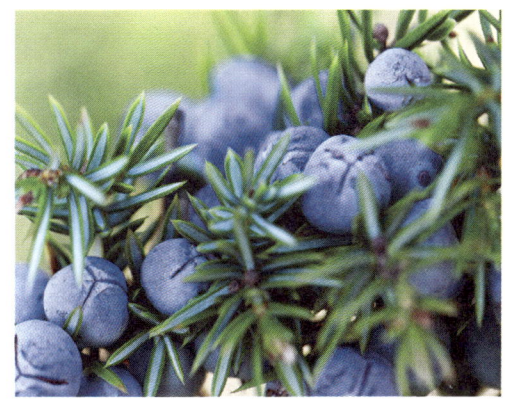

purposes. It was often burned in public places and homes to ward off plagues and other contagious diseases. The French recognized its disinfectant qualities and burned juniper, rosemary, and thyme in hospital wards to reduce airborne infections. Juniper is a common botanical ingredient that imparts its distinctive aroma to gin.

Main Qualities
Body/Skin

It reduces water retention before menstruation. It is included in cellulite and detoxifying blends. It helps recover from hangovers. It is helpful with arthritis and rheumatism. It is a good tonic for oily or congested skin.

Mind/Emotions

It helps lift guilt, despondency, lack of self-worth, and feeling undeserving of love. It supports you in facing deep-seated issues with courage. It helps ease resistance, bringing hidden emotions to the surface for healing.

Spiritual

Cleanses the atmosphere of a room and assists in meditation.

Warning: Do not use it during pregnancy.

How To Use

Bath, compress, hair care, inhalation, massage, room fragrance, perfume, skincare.

Lemongrass (Cymbopogon Citratus)

Family: Poaceae | Perfumery note: top/middle | Aroma: slightly sweet citrus aroma

Lemongrass is a perennial grass native to tropical and subsoil regions of south eastern Asia and Africa. It is tall and aromatic and grows in dense clumps with stiff stems and slender, blade-like leaves. Some cultures refer to it as "fever grass" because it can reduce fever. Lemongrass is propagated through root division, planted in the rainy season, and is ready for harvest six to eight months later.

Main Qualities
Body/Skin

It's an excellent physical tonic. It boosts the parasympathetic nervous system, hastening recovery from illness. It stimulates glandular secretions and muscles to aid digestion. It could help with colitis, indigestion, and gastroenteritis. It is an effective skin toner for tightening open pores. It can be used for oily and acne-prone skin, but care should be taken since it can irritate skin. It should be used in very low percentages.

Mind/Emotions

Treats symptoms of jet lag, clearing the head and relieving fatigue.

How To Use

Bath, compress, skincare, massage, perfume, room fragrance.

● Marjoram (Origanum Marjorana)

Family: Labiatae | Perfumery note: middle | Aroma: warm, penetrating, herbaceous and spicy

This well-known herb, growing to about two feet in height, features highly aromatic leaves and small white flowers arranged in clusters. It's also known as *Marjorana hortensis* or knotted marjoram. The essential oil is obtained through steam distillation of the leaves and flowering tops. It's important not to confuse this oil with the Spanish "marjoram", a species of thyme that only qualified aromatherapists should use. The name "marjoram" comes from the Greek word meaning "joy of the mountain", possibly inspired by the beautiful carpets of herbs that grew on mountainsides. Roman and Greek traditions included crowning newlyweds with wreaths woven from marjoram for good fortune and long life. Centuries later, Louis XIV of France favoured marjoram, scenting his clothes and apartments daily with marjoram and nutmeg. The dried leaves and flowers can be used in potpourris or scented and sedative herb pillows. Marjoram was a fashionable fragrance in Europe before the introduction of more exotic Eastern perfumes. While Queen Elizabeth of Hungary's rejuvenating Hungary Water contained marjoram (among other ingredients), today, the herb is widely used in Italian cuisine and the production of perfumes and toiletries.

Main Qualities
Body/Skin

It can lower high blood pressure. When applied, it warms the skin and has a powerful antispasmodic action that can ease arthritis pains, cramped muscles, muscle spasms, and menstrual cramps.

Mind/Emotions

It can be blended with Clary Sage, especially for menstrual difficulties. Calming, slightly sedative action and can be effective against some migraines. Soothing and relaxing for those you feel hostile or withdrawn. It is good for those who find it hard to display emotions. Assists with obsessive thoughts to find release from persistent mental thoughts.

Warning: It can stimulate menstrual flow and thus should never be used during pregnancy.

How To Use

Bath, compress, inhalation, skincare, massage, room freshener.

🌿 Neem (Azadirachta Indica)

Family: Meliaceae | Perfumery note: middle/base | Aroma: pungent, heady

Neem oil, though technically not an essential oil, is derived from the seeds of the neem tree. It is a versatile and potent natural oil with a rich history of use in traditional medicine, particularly in the Indian subcontinent. The neem tree is often called "the village pharmacy" and has been revered for centuries for its wide array of health benefits and uses in gardening, personal care, and pest control.

This green gold oil is obtained through pressing or solvent extraction methods from the seeds of the neem tree. Because of its bitter taste and pungent odour, neem oil is a natural deterrent for pests, making it a favoured eco-friendly alternative to chemical pesticides in organic farming and gardening. In skincare, neem oil is cherished for its anti-inflammatory, antibacterial, and antifungal properties, making it a valuable ingredient in formulations to treat acne, psoriasis, eczema, and other skin conditions. Its high fatty acid content nourishes and moisturises the skin, promoting a glowing complexion.

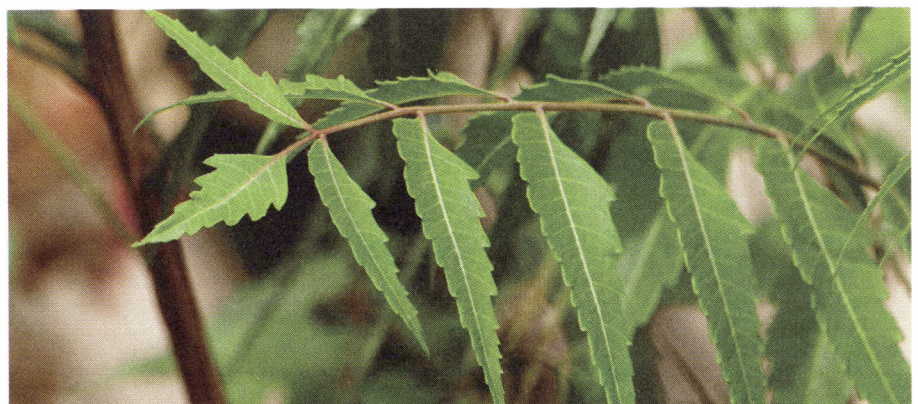

Main Qualities
Body/Skin

It helps significantly in relieving flatulence/removal of catarrhal matter and phlegm from the bronchial tubes. Used as an insecticide. It prevents hair fall and is good for hair growth. Destroys lice in the hair.

How To Use

Bath, compress, skincare, hair care, massage, room fragrance.

Palma Rosa (Cymbopogon martinii)

Family: Poaceae | Perfumery note: middle | Aroma: sharp, floral note with a hint of rose

Palmarosa, a member of the aromatic tropical grass family, originates from Central and North India but is now cultivated in Africa and Madagascar. This slender grass features panicles that bloom in a blue-white shade before ripening to a deep red. The essential oil, known for its fragrance, is distilled from the plant's leaves and flowers. Since the 18th century, palmarosa oil has been distilled, particularly in Turkey, as a cost-effective alternative or adulterant to the much more expensive Turkish rose oil.

Main Qualities
Body/Skin

It is effective in blends for treating various skin conditions as it helps balance sebum production, thus beneficial for extremely dry or oily skin. It blends beautifully with geranium, emphasises the scent of rose in any blend and works well with lavender. It tones dry and oily hair and is traditionally used in hair fall blends. It is good for acne and minor skin infections.

Mind/Emotions

It aids in releasing anger and grief. Useful as a PMS blend.

How To Use

Massage, room fragrance, skincare, bath, compress, skincare, hair care, massage, perfume.

Patchouli (Pogostemon Cablin)

Family: Labiatae | Perfumery note: middle/base | Aroma: warm, musty, an earthy, heavy scent

Patchouli is a plant that grows to about three feet high, with broad, furry leaves and white flowers tinged with purple. While native to Indonesia, patchouli oil is now produced in various regions, including Sumatra, India, the Philippines, and South America.

The essential oil of patchouli is obtained through the steam distillation of the plant's dried leaves. It is known for its rich, red-brown colour and thick consistency. Patchouli has a rich history of use in various cultures.

In the past, the Arabs, Chinese, and Japanese utilized patchouli for protection against infectious diseases. It also served as an antidote for snake and insect bites and addressing headaches, wounds, and diarrhoea. During the 19th century in India, powdered leaves of patchouli in little sachets were used to treat shawls for export, helping protect them from moths and insects during

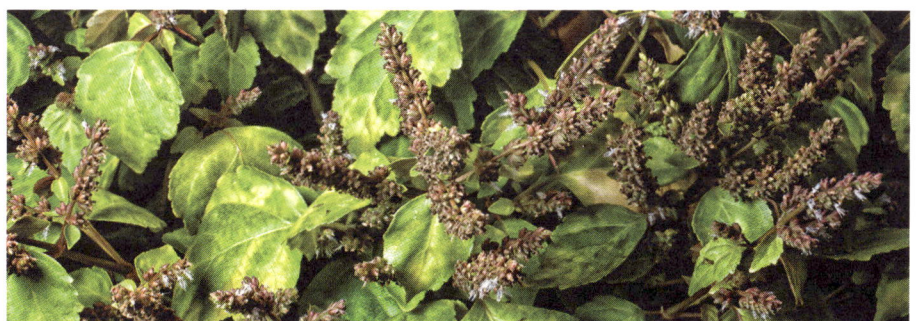

long voyages. Indian inks were once distinguished by their scent because they contained some patchouli; this helped fix the colour and make the ink dry quickly. In Europe, patchouli became fashionable, often blended with rose to create the well-known "patchouli" perfume. The oil's popularity experienced a revival in the 1960s when it was worn by hippies, becoming associated with peace and free love. Perfumers have long used patchouli as a natural fixative in Oriental fragrances, and it continues to be widely used in manufacturing cosmetics and toiletries.

Main Qualities
Body/Skin

It is an effective anti-inflammatory that helps heal cracked or inflamed skin, acne, dermatitis and eczema. It also tones and tightens the skin and is used in many anti-wrinkle blends. It helps regulate oily skin and dandruff and is very effective at combating cellulite.

Mind/Emotions

It is an excellent base note for perfume blends and is generally considered an aphrodisiac. It has a mildly sedative effect in small quantities and may be stimulating in large quantities.

How To Use

Bath, hair care, insect repellent, massage, perfume, room fragrance, skincare.

Peppermint (Mentha Piperita)

Family: Labiatae | Perfumery note: top | Aroma: cool, refreshing, penetrating menthol scent.

Peppermint is one of the most commonly used varieties of mint in aromatherapy, growing to a height of about three feet. Peppermint essential

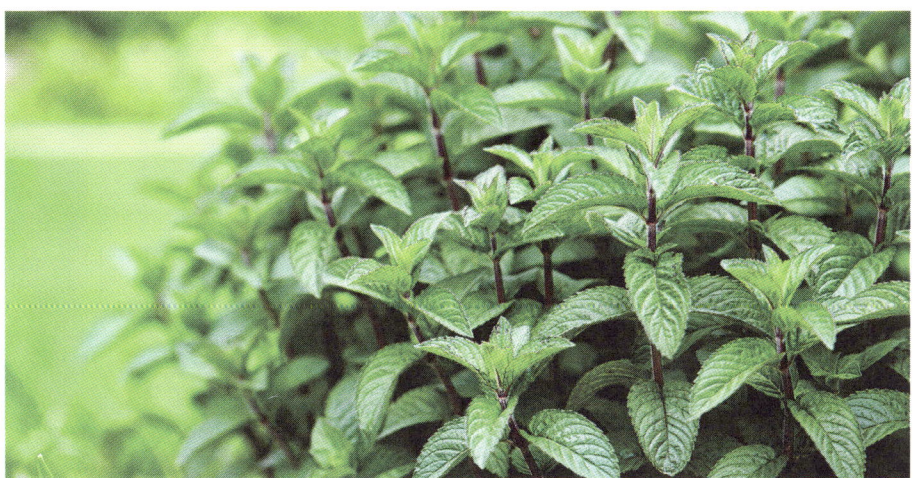

oil is obtained through steam distillation of its leaves and flowering tops. While believed to be native to southern Europe, it is now cultivated worldwide. The United States is the leading producer of peppermint oil, but English peppermint oil is often considered superior in quality.

Mint has a rich history of use in various cultures for its culinary and medicinal properties. The ancient Egyptians, Chinese and Japanese, as well as the Romans and Greeks, recognized its value. Mint was enjoyed in food and beverages and was even used as a refreshing addition to perfumes. Greek athletes applied mint to their muscles before competitions. In modern times, peppermint tea made from dried mint leaves is a popular beverage for its digestive benefits.

Mint is also widely used in the flavouring and fragrance industries, adding its refreshing essence to a range of products from food and drinks to toothpaste and toiletries. Considering its invigorating and revitalising qualities, mint's association with "eternal refreshment" is fitting. Peppermint is one of the "basic necessities" for a first aid kit.

Main Qualities
Body/Skin

It is often recommended for easing migraines (especially those stemming from digestive problems). It helps clear congestion in the sinuses. Peppermint is the ideal remedy for all digestive disorders, including nausea and vomiting. In a massage, it helps stimulate the lymph system.

Mind/Emotions

It clears the brain, helps concentration and is restorative in cases of mental fatigue.

How To Use

Bath, compress, insect repellent, massage, mouthwash, room fragrance, skin-care, steam inhalation.

Petitgrain (Citrus Aurantium)

Family: Rutaceae |Perfumery note: top/middle |Aroma: sharp, green.

Petitgrain essential oil is derived from the leaves and twigs of the bitter orange tree, also known as *Citrus vulgaris, bigaradia,* or Seville orange. This tree also provides neroli oil from its fragrant blossoms and bitter orange oil from the rind of its fruit. The bitter orange tree is originally native to China and the Middle East but has spread to various regions, including Mediterranean, Brazil and USA, where it is cultivated. The name "petitgrain" has a long history and originates from when oil was distilled from the unripe fruits of the bitter orange tree. In French, these small, unripe fruits were known as "petits grains", which translates to "little grains" in English. However, this method of oil extraction was found to be wasteful, and today, only the leaves and twigs of the tree are used to produce this fragrant oil. Petitgrain oil is currently widely used in the manufacture of bath oils, cosmetics and soaps and is a major component in high-quality eau de cologne.

Main Qualities
Body/Skin

It has a toning and astringent effect on the skin, refreshing a tired complexion and combating oiliness.

Mind/Emotions

Powerful oil that calms anxiety and panic, acting as an antidepressant. It tends to be a sedative, which agrees with its relaxing effect on the mind. It is recommended for treating rapid heartbeat and for insomnia.

How To Use

Bath, compress, skincare, hair care, massage, perfume, room fragrance.

Pine (Pinus Longifolia)

Family: Pinaceae | Perfumery note: top/middle | Aroma: light, fresh, woody

Pine *(Pinus sylvestris)* is a favoured variety of pine for aromatherapy. This majestic evergreen tree can grow to approximately fifteen feet and is primarily found in northern Europe and USA. The essential oil is obtained through the distillation of its needles. Additionally, this tree produces edible pine kernels that come from its cones. Pine kernels have been used as a source of nutrition for centuries, with recorded evidence of their use in ancient Egypt dating back to 1 AD. Native American Indians used pine needles to create extracts to act as a disinfectant and repel insects. Pine resin was used to address respiratory issues, and they even chewed gum made from pine resin to relieve stomach upsets. Today, the fragrance of pine is primarily in demand for bath oils and various toiletries. Once very common in Scotland, early man destroyed many trees.The tall, straight trunks were a favourite source of masts for sailing ships, as the trees can grow to thirty six m (120 ft) in height. Pine kernels or nut husks were found beside Roman dwellings excavated in Britain; seemingly,

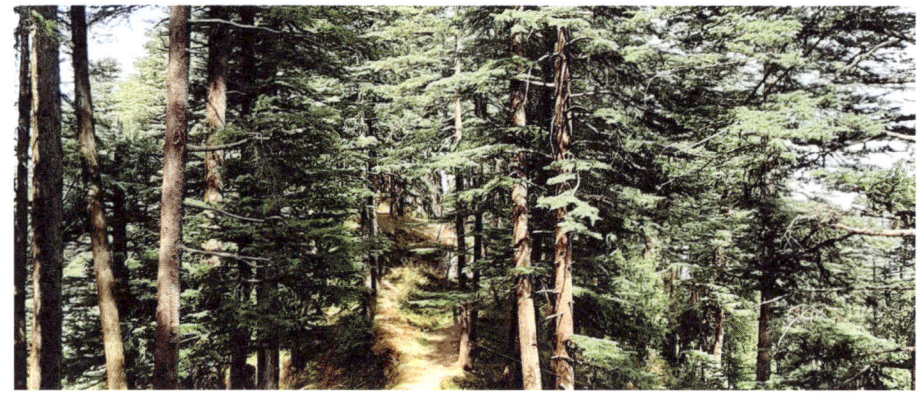

they were used for food and medicine. Pine cones can be used for yellowish dyes or aromatic fire kindling. Pine needle pillows can be made to help with breathing problems such as catarrh. The oil is used in many soaps, bath preparations, disinfectants, and detergents.

Main Qualities
Body/Skin

Excellent antiseptic, anti-fungal, and detoxifier. Use it in a sauna, two drops per pint of water. It enters the body through inhalation and expels toxins through perspiration. A few drops of pine and either lemon or eucalyptus in a scrub cleanses all surfaces, aiding in the elimination of unwanted bacteria and fungi on floors, in the tub, etc. It's a good addition to any cleaning mix. Pine is an excellent expectorant for cough, cold, and congestion, helping release mucus and ease breathing. It can help clear congestion in the sinuses, lungs, and bronchial passages.

Mind/Emotions

Enlivens the physical and mental spirit like a stroll through a pine forest. *Warning: Pine oil can be irritating to the skin. It should preferably be used in a diffuser to avoid contact with the skin. Those with allergies should avoid usage.*

How To Use

Bath, compress, insect repellent, room fragrance, steam inhalation.

Rosemary (Rosemarinus Officinalis)

Family: Labiatae | Perfumery note: top/middle | Aroma: fresh, camphor-like, herbal

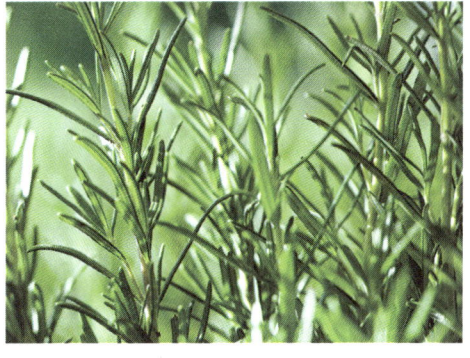

Rosemary is a versatile herb that can reach around four feet, featuring delicate needle-like leaves, dark on top and paler beneath, and small blue flowers. Its essential oil is extracted through steam distillation of the leaves and flowering tops. While rosemary is native to the Mediterranean region, it is now cultivated globally. The primary oil-exporting countries include France, Spain, and North Africa. Rosemary has enjoyed a rich history of culinary and medicinal use spanning centuries. The Romans held this herb in great reverence, considering it sacred. They used rosemary in various customs, such as gifting it to newlyweds and placing it on graves as a symbol of remembrance and friendship. Rosemary was often used in bouquets and scattered on house floors, where its scent would purify the surroundings. According to the English herbalist Bankes, merely smelling rosemary leaves could help keep one youthful. In addition to its various uses, rosemary played a part in creating Hungary Water, a perfume that made a Queen of Hungary so youthful that she, although aged seventy two, managed to woo the King of Poland! Even today, rosemary remains a prized ingredient in high-quality eau de cologne and many other toiletries. Its delightful fragrance is also a key component in the recognisable scent of vermouth.

Main Qualities
Body/Skin

In massage oil, it stimulates circulation and is used in blends for cellulite and oedema. Useful in blends to ease muscular and joint pain. Combats acne, dandruff, alopecia, and oily skin in cosmetics and soaps. A drop added to shampoo makes dark hair glow and may stimulate hair growth.

Mind/Emotions

Clearing and stimulating for feelings of disorientation, indecision, lethargy, feelings of inadequacy, feeling overwhelmed with responsibilities; known for its ability to wake up the body and spirit.

Warning: Avoid using during pregnancy and if you have high blood pressure or have a diagnosed seizure disorder.

How To Use

Bath, compress, hair care, insect repellent, room fragrance, skincare, steam inhalation.

Tea Tree (Melaleuca Alternifolia)

Family: Myrtaceae | Perfumery note: top/middle | Aroma: penetrating, camphor like, with a hint of spice

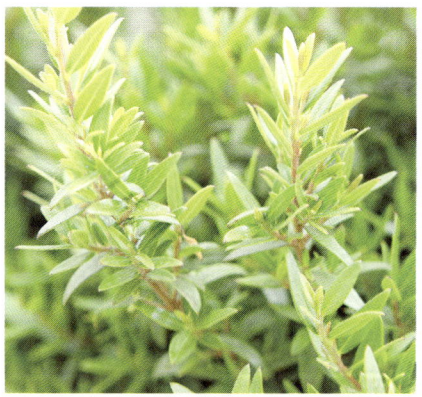

Tea tree is a shrub or small tree from which essential oil is extracted by distilling its fine needle-like leaves. It acquired its name when Captain Cook's sailors used it to brew a tea substitute. It has a rich history of traditional use among Aboriginal tribes in Australia, where it was considered a versatile remedy for preventing infections and promoting wound healing. Early European settlers in New South Wales used it as a bush remedy, particularly when medical supplies were scarce. However, it wasn't until the 1920s that scientific research began to investigate the medicinal potential of tea tree oil. In 1925, experiments confirmed that tea tree oil possessed remarkable antiseptic properties, being thirteen times stronger than carbolic acid. This discovery marked a significant turning point in understanding the therapeutic benefits of tea tree oil. In 1990, controlled experiments in Australia compared tea tree oil to benzoyl peroxide, a common acne treatment. The results demonstrated that tea tree oil was an effective alternative with fewer and less severe side effects. Tea tree oil is widely used in various fields, including dentistry. It can be found in numerous products, such as disinfectants, shampoos, and toothpaste, owing to its potent antiseptic properties. Tea tree has won a reputation as a "cure-all" essential oil.

Main Qualities
Body/Skin

Powerful anti-fungal, antiviral, and antibacterial properties; first suggestion for athlete's foot, nail viruses, and other fungal infections. Used in anti-acne remedies and diffusers to combat flu and other viral infections. Recommended as a remedy for vaginal candida infection. Distinct affinity for skin and fights dandruff.

How To Use

Bath, compress, hair care, room fragrance, skincare, steam inhalation.

🌟 SPICE

Extracted from seeds, bark, or roots of spices, these oils are warm and invigorating. Spicy essential oils are frequently used to boost energy, improve circulation, and add warmth to blends used in massage, diffusers, and personal care products.

🌶 Black Pepper (Piper Nigrum)

Family: Piperaceae | Perfumery note: top/middle | Aroma: pungent and spicy, like fresh peppercorns

Originating from the East, this shrub can reach heights of up to twenty feet when growing wild. The essential oil is meticulously extracted through steam distillation from the unripened dried fruit, commonly referred to as black peppercorn. Even as far back as the 5th century, the Romans recognized the digestive properties of black pepper. Gibbon, in his writings, tells us that black pepper was a favoured ingredient in the most extravagant Roman cuisine. Its value was so esteemed that it was sometimes used in place of money to pay rent or taxes. In his 17th-century book on herbs, astrologer-physician Nicholas Culpeper extolled the virtues of black pepper, stating that it dissolves gas in the stomach or bowels, promotes urination, eases coughs, and aids in treating various ailments of the chest. It was also a key component of potent antidotes. Black pepper has been imported to Europe from India and the East since the Middle Ages, primarily for its culinary appeal. Today, it continues to enjoy widespread use.

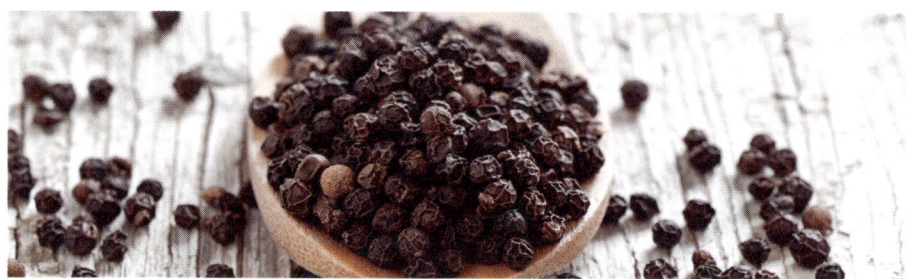

Main Qualities
Body/Skin

Pepper is one of the most stimulating oils. It is wonderful in a pre-sports rub to loosen muscles and a pain reliever for overworked muscles.

Types of Essential Oils

Mind/Emotions

It has a protective nature and helps clear away negative energies. It is said to increase self-confidence and fearlessness, encourage taking risks and listening to inner inspiration. It promotes endurance and flexibility, empowering you to act with confidence and accept outcomes.

Warning: Do not use it in high concentration, as it is a skin irritant.

How To Use

Bath, massage, room fragrance.

Cardamom (Elettaria Cardamomum)

Family: Zingiberaceae | Perfumery note: middle | Aroma: sweet, spicy

Cardamom, a tall perennial herb native to India and Sri Lanka, is renowned for its small seed pods, a coveted import in Europe, particularly the Mysore and Malabar varieties. Thriving in moist soil at altitudes of 600-1500 m, cardamom can be found both wild and cultivated. Its leaves are long and lance-shaped, with the plant producing a flowering and fruiting stem from its base. Mysore cardamom stems stand erect, while Malabar stems trail along the ground. The flowers, typically blooming in May, are yellowish with a purple lip, leading to ovoid fruit capsules by early October. These two cm long capsules split into three sections filled with dark brownish-red seeds. An interesting challenge in cardamom cultivation is the potential loss of pods to seed-loving gourmet lizards! Harvesting

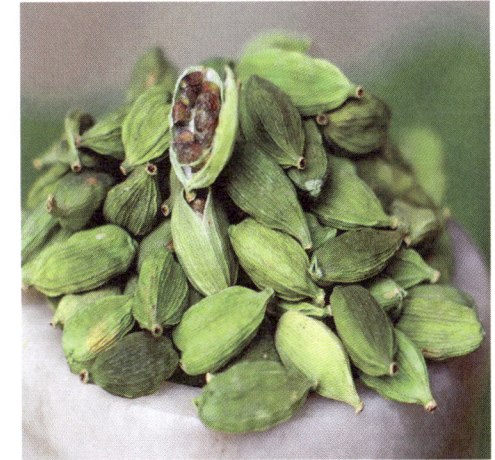

the pods just before full ripeness is crucial; otherwise, the seeds may burst open during drying, losing their essential oils and fragrance. Cardamom is the third most expensive spice globally, following saffron and vanilla. In India, its used as both a spice and a medicinal agent dating back over a thousand years, with references in Ayurvedic texts calling it "Ela". The essential oil of cardamom is extracted through steam distillation of these aromatic seeds. This essence is a liquid, primarily colourless with a slight yellowish-green hue, and is cherished for its warm, soft, and spicy fragrance, making it a popular choice in floral perfume compositions. In Indian cooking, cardamom pods are used whole or lightly crushed in curries and pilafs, and the ground seeds are a constituent of many masala powders. Cardamom also flavours sweets and sweet dishes in India. In Sweden, cardamom is used as a flavouring for cakes, breads, and pastries, as it is in Germany, other Scandinavian countries and some parts of Russia. Cardamom can be used in punches, hot spiced or mulled wines, or to flavour bedouin coffee.

Main Qualities
Body/Skin

Provides relief for menopausal symptoms and rheumatic stiffness in massage. Helps against urine retention and stomach disorders. Relieves flatulence and strengthens digestion. Excellent for respiratory diseases. An excellent expectorant. Used in toothpaste and syrup for pulmonary problems in France. The seeds can be coarsely ground and used in potpourris and herb pillows. The seeds are considered to be an aphrodisiac as well as a digestive aid after meals.

Mind/Emotions

It provides wisdom when feeling burdened and supports a generous spirit. It encourages openness and compassion, helping you extend friendship and support to others in need.

How To Use
Bath, compress, skincare, massage, perfume, room fragrance.

Cinnamon Bark (Cinnamomum Cassia)
Family: Lauraceae | Perfumery note: middle | Aroma: spicy, sweet

Cinnamon trees, known for their evergreen nature, can reach up to sixty feet, though they are more commonly found at heights between twenty and thirty feet. These trees feature shiny, ovoid leaves and bear tiny yellow flowers and fruits, with the entire tree exuding a spicy scent. When they reach six to eight years old, their bark is harvested in long strips and dried under the sun. Both the bark and leaves are steam distilled to extract the essential oil. Originally native to Ceylon (Sri Lanka), cinnamon is now also cultivated in tropical regions like India, the Seychelles, and Mauritius. One of the oldest known spices, cinnamon, referred to as "ten-chu-kwei" or "cinnamon of India" in Emperor Shen Nung's treatise around 2700 BC and as "quesiah" in the Bible, has a rich history. The ancient Egyptians used it for embalming and to ward off epidemics. Arab traders initially kept its origin a secret while supplying it to the Greeks and Romans. The spice was so coveted that it drove the Portuguese to discover a sea route to India and Ceylon in the 16th century. The Dutch later took control of Ceylon in the mid-17th century, monopolising the cinnamon trade for about 150 years and initiating its systematic cultivation around 1770.

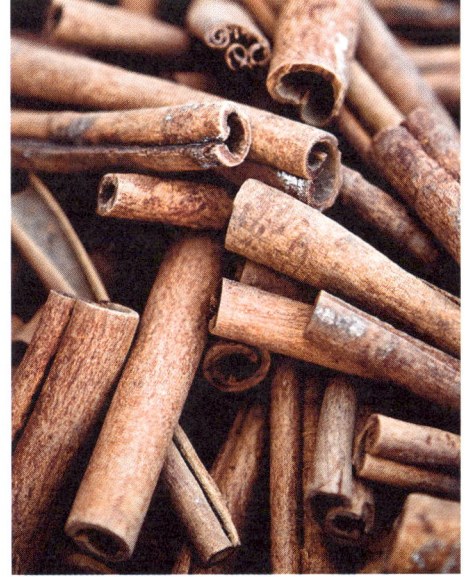

Main Qualities
Body/Skin

It is a good stimulant and helps in relieving flatulence. It helps to increase the secretion and discharge of urine. Prevents stress. Improves complexion. Good for common cold, influenza, and sore throat. Helps during excessive menstruation.

Mind/Emotions

Enhances sharpness of mind and brings joy.

How To Use

Bath, compress, skincare, massage, perfume, room fragrance.

Cinnamon Leaf (Cinnamomum Xeylanicum)

Family: Lauraceae | Perfumery Note: middle | Aroma: spicy, sweet

Cinnamon leaf essential oil, extracted from the leaves of the tree, is a potent and aromatic oil. Revered for centuries, this oil has a rich history that traces back to ancient Egypt. Egyptians used it in embalming rituals, believing its potent aroma could ward off evil spirits and preserve the body for the afterlife. The spice's popularity spread to ancient Greece and Rome, where it was used for its therapeutic properties and as a luxury item in perfumery and incense. In medieval Europe, cinnamon was a sought-after spice, contributing to the prosperity of the spice trade. During this time, explorers like Vasco da Gama and Christopher Columbus set out on expeditions to find direct trade routes to Asia, driven by the lucrative potential of spices.

Main Qualities
Body/Skin

A powerful antiseptic, it effectively stops the spread of coughs, colds, and viral infections. Topically, cinnamon generally alleviates aches, pains, and stiffness in the muscles and joints and enhances circulation.

How To Use

Bath, compress, skincare, massage, perfume, room fragrance.

🌿 Clove (Syzygium Aomaticum)

Family: Myrtaceae | Perfumery note: middle | Aroma: spicy, sharp

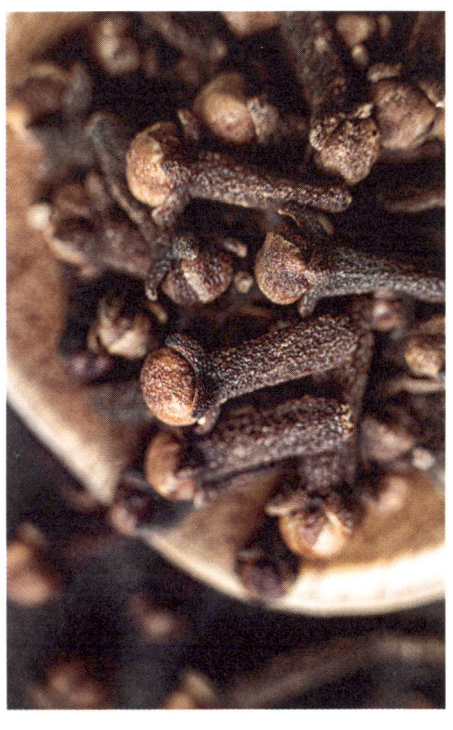

Clove essential oil is derived from the flower buds of the *Syzygium aromaticum* tree. Known for its rich, spicy aroma and warming characteristics, it is native to the Maluku Islands in Indonesia, where parents planted a clove tree when a child was born. When the clove forests were first discovered, all were enchanted with the fragrance and beauty of this tropical evergreen tree that "must always see the sea" in order to thrive.

Cloves were highly prized in ancient China, where they were used as a breath freshener for court officials before they spoke to the emperor. The spice has a high value, making it a coveted commodity in the spice trade, leading to intense competition among traders. Cloves reached India by 1700 BC and southern Europe by the 1st century AD. Arab traders introduced cloves to Europe in the 4th century, where they were used in the Middle Ages to mask the taste of poorly preserved food. Medieval Europe saw cloves as a symbol of luxury and wealth and used to flavour foods and wines, as well as for medicinal purposes.

Main Qualities
Body/Skin

It is stimulating, carminative, a strong germicide and antiseptic, and helps relieve flatulence. It is also a good stimulant for digestion and metabolism and helps relieve toothaches.

Mind/Emotions

Helps to set firm boundaries and break free from toxic patterns. It empowers you to stand up for yourself with confidence and compassion. Ideal for reinforcing your ability to say no, articulate your needs, and foster healthy relationships.

How To Use

Bath, compress, skincare, massage, perfume, room fragrance.

❋ Coriander Seed (Coriandrum Sativum)

Family: Umbeliferae | Perfumery note: middle | Aroma: sweet, herbaceous, spicy, woody

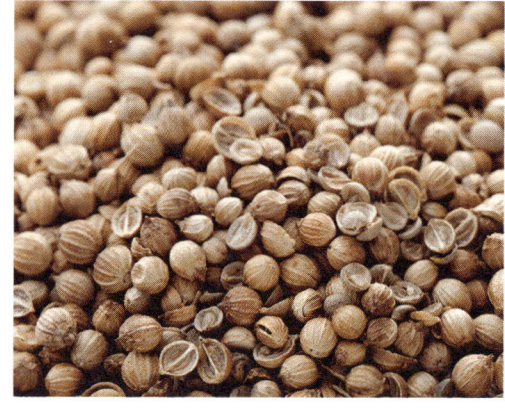

Coriander derives its name from the Greek word 'koris' for bug and is thought to have a scent reminiscent of bed bugs, particularly in its young leaves. This umbelliferous plant is native to Southern Europe, North Africa, South America, and Russia. It features bright green leaves deeply indented at the base, resembling continental parsley, and become feathery higher on the plant. Coriander blooms with umbels of mauve flowers that eventualy produce seeds that are utilized in cooking and seasoning. As one of the potentialy oldest flavourings known, coriander's use spans several cultures and eras. In ancient Egypt, its seeds were crushed into bread dough, and its essential oil was used for religious rites. The Bible mentions it as one of the bitter herbs to be consumed during Passover, and in India, it served both culinary and magical purposes, including invocations to the gods. Coriander has been historically considered an aphrodisiac, and the Greeks and Romans recognized its stimulant, digestive, and carminative effects. In a herb distillery, a mishap led to the spillage of fifty litres of coriander oil across the cement floor. Despite the efforts of eight workers, the oil seeped into every nook, creating an overpowering atmosphere. Initially, the workers found humour in the situation, laughing and joking. However, their moods shifted to aggression, and the intoxicating fumes even caused physical fights and extreme nausea. The affected employees were eventually sent home to recover from their subsequent extreme fatigue. This incident highlighted the potent effects of concentrated coriander oil exposure.

Main Qualities
Body/Skin

Coriander can stimulate appetite, ease indigestion, and relieve neuralgia. It strengthens the stomach and helps relieve flatulence. It increases urine discharge and reduces fever as well. It is helpful as an antispasmodic and anti-inflammatory. It's a good addition to rubs for aching muscles. It is good for the flu, as it is antibacterial and can be used as a chest rub.

Mind/Emotions

The scent is warm, welcoming and relaxing, although, like other spices, it is usually listed as a stimulant.

How To Use

Bath, compress, massage, perfume, room fragrance.

✿ Curry Leaf (Murraya Koenigii)

Family: Rutaceae | Perfumery note: middle | Aroma: spicy, bitter

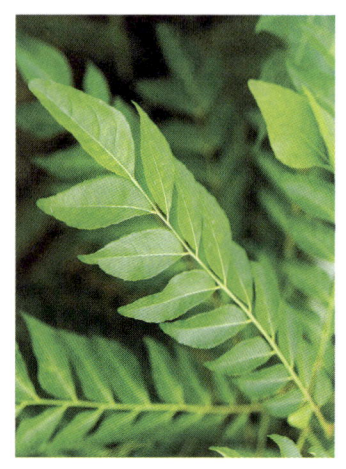

Curry leaf essential oil is extracted from the leaves of the *Murraya koenigii* tree and can grow to about twenty feet tall. Native to India and Sri Lanka, the curry leaf tree has long been revered in traditional Ayurvedic and Siddha medicine for its therapeutic properties. Curry leaves were used to treat various ailments, from digestive issues to skin conditions. In Indian cuisine, curry leaves are an essential ingredient, adding a rich, aromatic flavour to dishes. The leaves were also used in ancient rituals and ceremonies, symbolising purification and protection. Curry leaf tree, often found growing in backyards and gardens across India, is more than just a culinary staple. It holds a significant place in the cultural and spiritual lives of the people.

Main Qualities
Body/Skin

It strengthens the function of the stomach and acts as a mild laxative. It prevents diabetes and problems due to hereditary factors like premature greying and helps in nourishing hair roots. Excellent oil to stimulate hair growth and retain natural pigmentation.

How To Use

Bath, compress, massage, perfume, room fragrance.

✿ Fennel Seed (Foeniculum Vulgare)

Family: Umbelliferae | Perfumery note: middle | Aroma: herbaceous, light and sweet, reminiscent of aniseed

The fennel plant features delicate leaves and clusters of small yellow flowers. Essential oil is derived through steam distillation of powdered seeds. In aromatherapy, the preferred choice is sweet fennel (variety dulce), also known as Roman or French fennel. Bitter fennel (variety amara) contains toxic oil and should never be used. 'Fennel' originates from the Latin 'foenum', meaning 'hay'. Ancient Egyptians used fennel for its believed medicinal properties, harnessing it for various purposes. Different civilisations, including the Greeks and Romans, valued its purifying qualities. Pliny, the Roman author, attributed more than twenty medicinal uses to fennel, and in the Middle Ages, it was thought to ward off evil spirits and bad luck. Sprigs of fennel were often hung over entrances. Fennel tea is known for its ability to settle the stomach, relieve nausea, promote milk flow in nursing women, and aid digestion. This tradition even extended to feeding colicky horses fennel and dandelion leaves among Romany communities. Today, fennel is a common ingredient in many proprietary medicines, particularly cough mixtures and gripe water for infants.

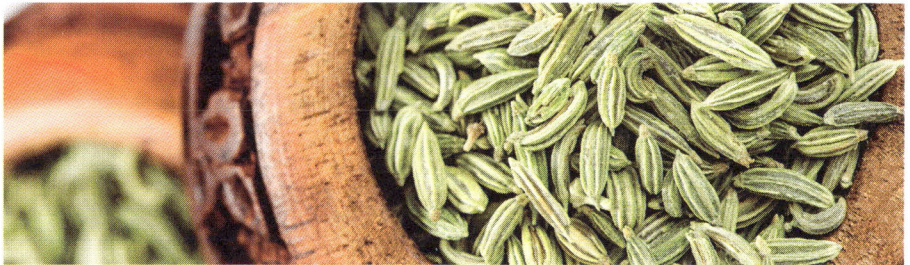

Main Qualities
Body/Skin

Fennel is recommended for massage for cellulite, indigestion, and gas. It is also useful for PMS and menstrual difficulties. It detoxifies the body from overindulgence in alcohol, nicotine, and other toxic substances. Fennel is often recommended for breast-firming massage and promoting milk flow in nursing women.

Mind/Emotions

It eases stress and nervous tension without having the mildly sedative effect that many relaxing essential oils bring.

Warning: Fennel can be a skin irritant. Do not use it on young children, during pregnancy, or if you suffer from epilepsy.

How To Use

Bath, compress, massage, perfume, room fragrance, skincare.

Fenugreek (Trigonella Foenum Graecum)

Family: Fabaceae | Perfumery note: middle/base | Aroma: warm, woody

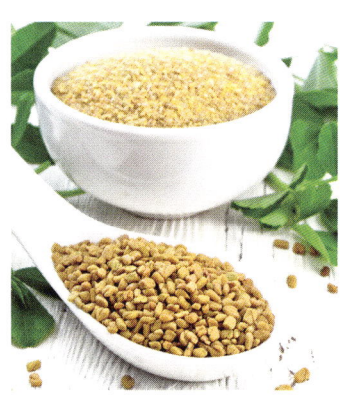

Fenugreek is one of the oldest healing plants, originating in central Asia around 4000 BC. Its leaves consist of three small obovate to oblong leaflets, and the oil is extracted from the seeds through steam distillation. It has a warming and soothing effect, making it beneficial for massage blends to relieve muscle pain. It's also used in aromatherapy for its comforting and grounding aroma, which can help reduce stress and promote relaxation. It was used by the ancient Egyptians to embalm the dead and is mentioned in ancient medical books. Fenugreek oil has also been found in the tomb of Tutankhamun. Fenugreek has been used in Indian cuisine for 3,000 years for its nutty flavour. Its seeds and leaves are common ingredients in dishes from the Indian subcontinent.

Main Qualities
Body/Skin

It helps in alleviating swelling and pain. Increases secretion and discharge of urine. Relieves flatulence. It enables the body to detoxify. It helps remove dandruff, stimulates hair growth, and preserves the natural colour while keeping hair silky.

How To Use

Bath, compress, skincare, massage, perfume, room fragrance.

Ginger (Zingiber Officinale)

Family: Zingiberaceae | Perfumery note: middle/base | Aroma: sharp, spicy

Ginger, a tropical herbaceous perennial, stands out with its elongated, spiky leaves resembling reeds and yellow flowers with a purple lip reminiscent of orchids. However, what truly sets ginger apart is its underground rhizomes or tubers, often branching out like fingers and referred to as "hands", which are harvested for their spice. Believed to have originated in India, ginger was among the first spices transported to Europe from Asia. The Spanish conquistadors introduced ginger to the West Indies, where it rapidly became naturalised, particularly in Jamaica, 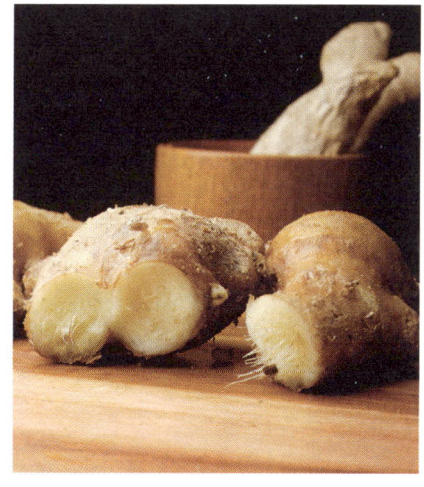 which emerged as a leading producer. Today, ginger is cultivated in several countries with favourable climates, including India accounting for half of the global production Malaysia, Africa, Japan (home to forty species), China, Queensland, and Florida. For centuries, ginger has been prized in India, China, and Japan for its culinary applications and medicinal benefits, playing a significant role in the traditional cuisines of these regions.

Types of Essential Oils

Main Qualities
Body/Skin

It is wonderful in massage blends for aching joints, muscles, indigestion, and gas. Its heat can irritate the skin, so be sure to dilute it. It is a warming ingredient in a "chest rub" for a cold or flu. It also works wonders for a sore throat. It can be an aphrodisiac and has been used to treat male impotence.

How To Use

Inhalation, bath, compress, skincare, hair care, massage, perfume, room fragrance.

Nutmeg (Myristica Fragrans)

Family: Myristicaceae | Perfumery note: middle | Aroma: warm, sweet

Nutmeg trees, majestic evergreens, originate from the Moluccas and areas capable of reaching heights between eighteen to twenty four meters (sixty to eighty feet), They display a unique botanical feature: they are dioecious, meaning individual trees are either male or female. A typical plantation setup involves one male tree for every ten to twelve female trees, earning them the playful nickname of "harem trees". It takes nearly a decade, around eight or nine

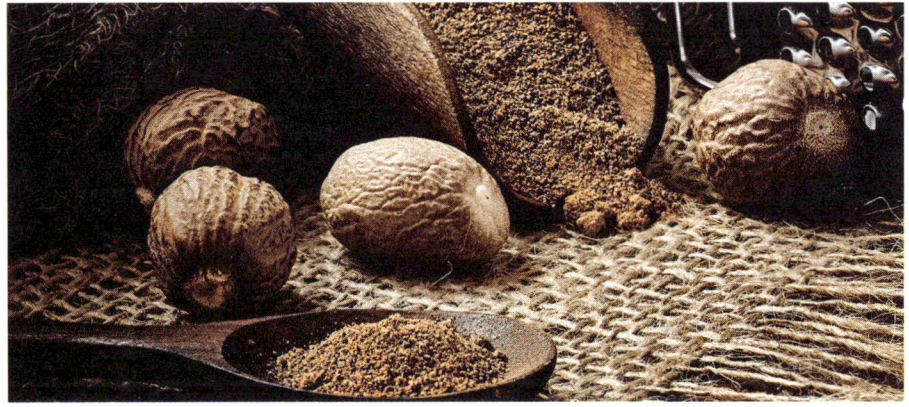

years, for the trees to start flowering and fruiting, making early determination of their sex impossible. Initially, a mature tree might produce about 100 fruits. Still, as it reaches the age of thirty, its productivity can surge to an impressive 3,000 to 4,000 fruits annually, with a potential productive lifespan of up to seventy years. The transplantation of nutmeg trees to the West Indies during the British Empire's tenure in the Moluccas marked the beginning of a thriving nutmeg industry outside their native soil. These islands, especially Grenada, have become synonymous with high-quality nutmeg production, celebrating the tree's rich heritage and significant role in the global spice trade. The journey of the nutmeg fruit to maturity is a spectacle of nature, starting with yellowish blossoms that give way to large fruits resembling yellow apricots or plums. As these fruits ripen, they eventually split open to unveil the treasure within a glossy black seed, the nutmeg, elegantly encased in a vibrant red, lacy covering known as mace.

Main Qualities

It must be used cautiously as some authorities state it has psychotropic effects and is a hallucinogen.

Body/Skin

It is an excellent digestive stimulant for those who cannot digest food and is a useful oil in treating nausea, vomiting, indigestion, etc. It is gently warming in a massage blend, and that, coupled with its anti-inflammatory characteristics, makes it helpful in treating sore joints and muscles and arthritis.

Mind/Emotions

It is invigorating and stimulating. Helps to clear away debris we no longer need. *Warning: Please avoid during pregnancy and use with care.*

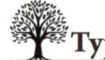 Saffron (Crocus Sativus)

Family: Iridaceae | Perfumery note: middle | Aroma: sweet, floral, earthy

Saffron is referred to as the "King of Spices" and "Red Gold" and is a highly prized spice derived from the stigmas of the *Crocus sativus* flower, a member of the iris family. Cultivated for over 3,500 years in the Middle East and the Mediterranean region, saffron has a rich history that spans cultures, continents, and civilisations. Its vibrant crimson threads are notable for their unique, delicate flavour and colouring properties and impressive health benefits. The cultivation and harvest of saffron require meticulous care and labour-intensive processes, contributing to its status as one of the world's most expensive spices by weight. Each *Crocus sativus* flower produces only three stigmas, which must be handpicked during a short annual flowering season and carefully dried. It takes approximately 75,000 saffron flowers to produce a single pound of saffron spice, highlighting the intensive effort required for its production. Saffron's distinct taste and aroma are slightly sweet, floral, and earthy and lead to versatile use in dishes worldwide, from Spanish paella and Italian risotto to Iranian saffron rice and Indian biryani. Beyond its culinary uses, saffron has been utilized in traditional medicine for centuries, owing to its potential health benefits. It is believed to possess antioxidant, anti-inflammatory, and antidepressant properties, and research suggests it may aid in improving mood, enhancing cognitive function, and supporting heart health.

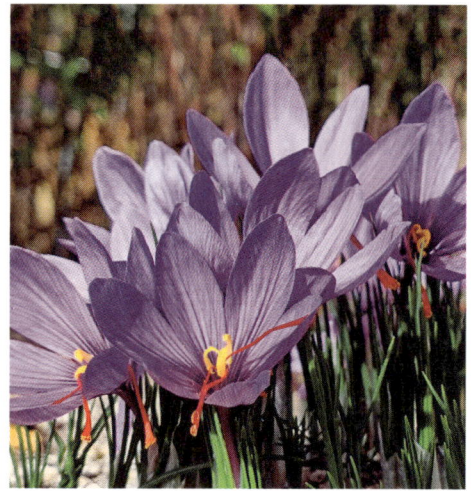

In addition to its health benefits, saffron has been used in textiles as a dye and in perfumery for its unique fragrance. Its historical significance is evident in ancient manuscripts, and it has been revered in various cultures for its medicinal properties and as a symbol of wealth and prosperity.

Main Qualities
Body/Skin

Strengthens and promotes the functioning of the stomach. Good stimulant and boosts libido.

How To Use

Bath, compress, skincare, massage, perfume, room fragrance.

Turmeric (Curcuma Longa)

Family: Zingiberaceae | Perfumery note: middle/ base | Aroma: herbaceous, spicy

Turmeric, a golden-yellow spice, has been a staple in culinary, medicinal, and cultural traditions for thousands of years, primarily in South Asia and the Middle East. It was first cultivated in the Indian subcontinent, where it has been an integral part of Ayurvedic medicine due to its potent anti-inflammatory and antioxidant properties. Historical records suggest that turmeric was used for cooking, as a dye, and in religious ceremonies. Its active ingredient, curcumin, is believed to offer numerous health benefits and is recognized and utilized in various traditional medicine systems worldwide. The spice made its way along the Spice Routes to Europe and Africa, becoming valued for its flavour and health-giving properties. Turmeric heals the skin of minor infections and blemishes and detoxifies it, keeping it healthy without reducing its natural sebum, making it a popular ingredient in skincare products. In Indian marriages, a special ritual revolves around turmeric or haldi—there is singing, dancing, and music played while family members scrub down the

Types of Essential Oils

bride and groom with turmeric to cleanse and rid the skin of minor issues and to help de-tan, resulting in clear and glowing skin. Today, turmeric continues to be celebrated globally, not just as a culinary ingredient but also for its therapeutic potential, underpinning its historical significance with modern scientific research.

Main Qualities
Body/Skin

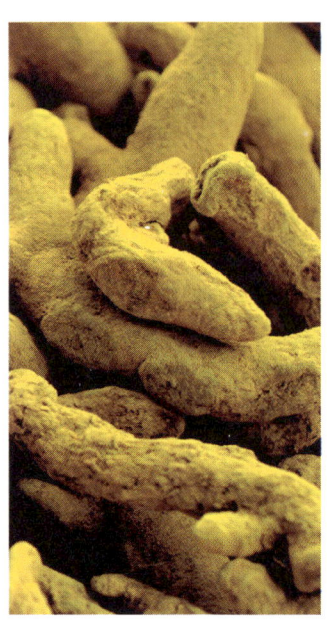

Cleans and disinfects skin without drying out the natural oils. Cures skin ulcers. Bactericidal and antiallergenic qualities have an inflammatory effect and are helpful in arthritis. It strengthens the stomach's action, promotes its action as a tonic, and acts as a blood purifier. It relieves flatulence and acts as a stimulant and a tonic. Antiseptic and good for chronic cough and throat irritations. It promotes discharge from the nose and offers quicker relief from congestion and cold problems.

HOW TO USE

Bath, compress, skincare, hair care, massage, perfume, room fragrance.

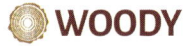 WOODY

Sourced from tree bark, wood, roots, sap, or resin, these oils have deep, rich scents and grounding properties. Woody essential oils are often used in meditation and relaxation and to create a sense of inner peace in diffusers, incense, and body oils.

Camphor (Cinnamomum Camphora)

Family: Lauraceae | Perfumery note: top | Aroma: cooling, pungent

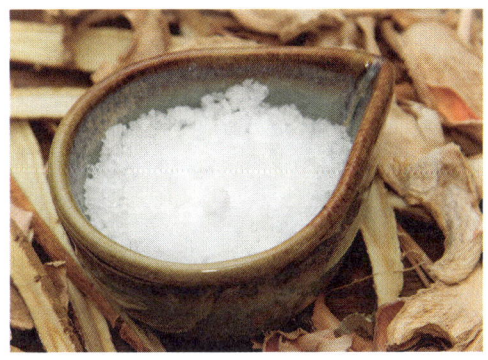

Camphor, a crystalline substance with a cooling, pungent aroma, is derived from the *Cinnamomum camphora* tree. This tree, a member of the laurel or bay family, is native to China, Taiwan and Japan and has also been cultivated in Sri Lanka and California. The camphor tree can reach over thirty meters in height and is known for its massive trunk and long lifespan, with some Chinese records claiming it has lived up to 1,000 years. Camphor has been highly valued in traditional medicine for centuries. In Ayurveda, it's used for various conditions, including eye injuries and headaches, and as a tonic. Chinese medicine has utilized it for over 2,000 years. Its rarity once made it more valuable than gold in Europe, where Avicenna first noted it in the 11th century. French researchers have studied its potential as a cardiac tonic, sexual stimulant, analgesic for rheumatism, and antiseptic for pulmonary infections. It is important to note that borneol camphor should not be used alongside homoeopathic remedies, as it can counteract their effects.

Main Qualities
Body/Skin

It is used as an antiseptic to disinfect rooms and during epidemics. It is most commonly used in vapours and liniments for colds, chills, and inflammatory conditions. Camphor is slightly cold to the touch. It is used locally to numb the peripheral sensory nerves as a counter-irritant in rheumatism and sprains in inflammatory conditions.

Mind/Emotions

Encourages upliftment and stimulation. Also helps clear negative energies from a space and clears the aura.

How To Use

Bath, compress, massage, room fragrance, skincare preparations.

Cedarwood (Cedrus Deodara)

Family: Pinaceae | Perfumery note: base | Aroma: soft, warm, woody

The Deodar cedarwood tree, a majestic species native to the Himalayan region, stands as the tallest among cedars, with some specimens soaring over 200 feet. Deriving its name from the Sanskrit 'devadāru', which translates to 'wood of the gods', Cedrus deodara is an imposing evergreen tree. It is distinguished by its large, dioecious structure, yellow-green needles, and upward-reaching branches. Historically, Cedarwood has held significant religious and cultural roles, particularly in Hindu traditions. It was commonly utilized in constructing temples and palaces and often planted in sacred groves near temples. Hindu myths frequently reference this tree, highlighting its spiritual significance. Cedarwood's wood, known for its aromatic qualities, is used in incense. The smoke from this wood served as a source of inspiration for female oracles in the Hindu Kush. Cedarwood was also used to induce trance, while in Native American culture, it is said to have the ability to counter negative forces. The temples of Solomon in Jerusalem were built with cedars from Lebanon, and it is possible the Hebrews extracted oil from the wood. The tree also connects with ancient Egypt, as Queen Hatshepsut chose cedar to embellish her temple. In addition to its religious uses, Cedarwood has found applications in various domains such as medicine, perfumery, and cosmetics. Its natural properties, including insect repellence and durability, made it an ideal material for crafting sarcophagi, evidenced by archaeological findings in mummified remains. Beyond these uses, Cedarwood also provides quality plywood, which is a popular material for manufacturing pencils.

Main Qualities
Body/Skin

Excellent for easing the discomfort of any respiratory ailment. It can be used in a diffuser or added to a chest rub, often used as an expectorant, and in a blend to combat cellulite. It stimulates hair growth and is good for dandruff, dry hair, and alopecia. Good for acne and oily or dry skin. It can be used for blisters and eczema. Repels insects.

Mind/Emotions

Emotionally, it can calm anxiety, offering steadiness and hope and help to diffuse fear. Promotes restful sleep. Focuses attention when concentration is lacking forscattered thoughts, daydreaming, and living in the future. Purifies to aid in spiritual awakening.

Warning: It is to be avoided by people with high blood pressure or heart problems.

How To Use

Bath, compress, hair care, inhalation, massage, insect repellent, perfume, room fragrance, skincare.

Frankincense (Boswellia Carterii)

Family: Burseraceae | Perfumery note: middle/base | Aroma: woody, spicy with a slight pine-like top note.

Frankincense, a resilient shrub, thrives even in barren soil. Its origins trace back to the Middle East, but today, the oil is exported from North Africa, China, and western India. Deep incisions are made into the tree's trunk, from which white resinous matter exudes in large "tears", ovoid in shape.

These dry and fall to the ground, where they are collected. The tears are whitish-yellow, milky and waxy. Commercially, it is usually supplied in yellowish blocks covered with white dust; it is also available powdered. Frankincense has been prized since ancient times and featured prominently in spiritual rituals from China to Egypt. The ancient Egyptians blended frankincense with myrrh, juniper berries, cinnamon, mint, sweet flag, and raisins to create kyphi, a popular temple incense serving as a wine additive. Egyptians and Hebrews held frankincense in high regard, using it for various purposes, from fumigating homes to freshening breath and incorporating it into rejuvenating creams and face masks. In the past, frankincense was used for toothaches and respiratory and digestive ailments. Today, frankincense is used as incense in various religious traditions, including the Catholic Church and Buddhism.

Main Qualities
Body/Skin

It is excellent for asthma or chest congestion. It acts as an expectorant and clears congestion. Blending into facial creams or oils for ageing skin and scars is wonderful.

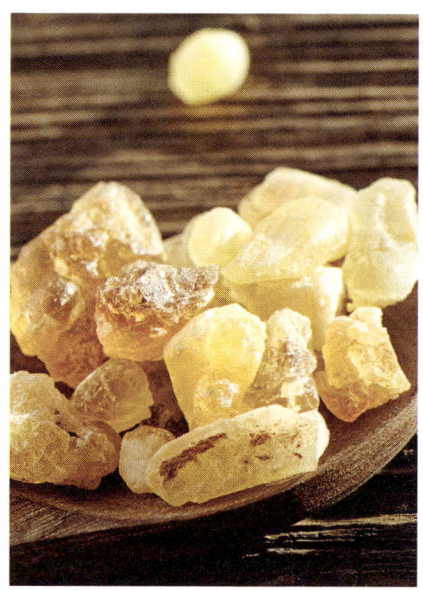

Mind/Emotions

Traditionally used for spiritual growth and meditation. It is believed to have a centring effect on emotions and helps you connect to Divine love. It helps promote sleep.

How To Use

Bath, compress, perfume, room fragrance, skincare, steam inhalation.

Sandalwood (Santalum Album)

Family: Santalaceae | Perfumery note: base | Aroma: subtle, warm, woody with a hint of spice

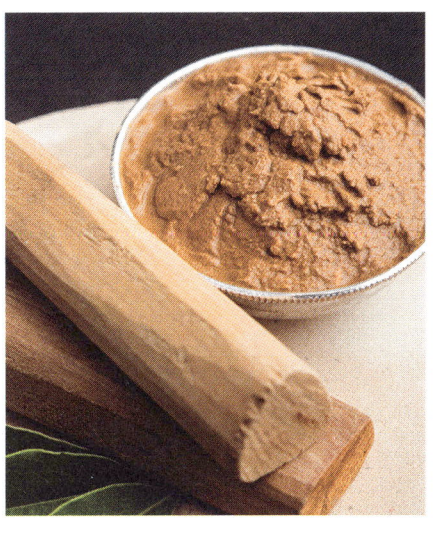

Sandalwood is an evergreen tree native to Asia. Its essential oil is derived from the heartwood, located at the very centre of the tree, through steam distillation. To make this process economically viable, the trees are alowed to mature for at least thirty years before they are harvested. While there are various types of sandalwood, such as Australian sandalwood *(Santalum spicatum)*, the oil from Mysore in India is widely regarded as superior for therapeutic purposes. Sandalwood has been revered for its divine fragrance since ancient times. It was used to create perfumes, cosmetics, and temple incense; in some cases, entire Hindu temples were constructed from the wood of the sandalwood tree. Ancient Egyptians imported sandalwood and used it in medicine, embalming, and ritual, burning it to venerate the gods. In Islamic tradition, luring goddess-like beings called the Houris were believed to be made of sandalwood in the afterlife. In ancient China, sandalwood was employed to address skin and digestive issues. Ayurvedic practitioners continue to use sandalwood to treat urinary and respiratory tract infections. Tahitian women have used a blend of sandalwood and coconut oils to condition their hair for generations. Traditionally, all attars were made with sandalwood as the base oil, but over time, with the rising wood prices, sandalwood was replaced with cheaper substitutes.

Main Qualities
Body/Skin

Tonic for the immune system. Often used to treat urinary tract problems. It balances dry and oily skin and is useful in treating acne, dry eczema, and soothing barber rash. Helps in anti-ageing blends.

Mind/Emotions

It is good for nervous tension, relaxes stress and irritability, and a leviates depression. It is an excelent balancing oil for people who are possessive, want their own way, and have difficulty forgiving. It is also an aphrodisiac, helpful for sexual anxiety.

Spiritual

Aids in meditation and spiritual growth.

How To Use

Bath, compress, perfume, room fragrance, skincare, steam inhalation.

Spikenard (Nardostachys Jatamasi)

Family: Caprifoliaceae | Perfumery note: base | Aroma: resinous, damp, warm

Woody Spikenard, a highly valued ancient aromatic plant, has deep roots in historical and religious contexts. This herb is native to the high altitudes of the Himalayan mountains. Recognizable by its pink, bell-shaped flowers, spikenard has been celebrated for its earthy, musky scent that is both soothing and grounding. It has been used for thousands of years in Ayurvedic medicine, traditional Chinese medicine, and by the ancient Egyptians, Greeks and Romans. Spikenard was considered extremely precious, used in religious ceremonies, and as perfume. It is most famously mentioned in the Bible where Mary Magdalene anointed Jesus' feet with costly spikenard oil, symbolising devotion and honour. Despite its ancient lineage, spikenard remains a cherished and revered oil in modern holistic practices for its unique scent and wide range of benefits.

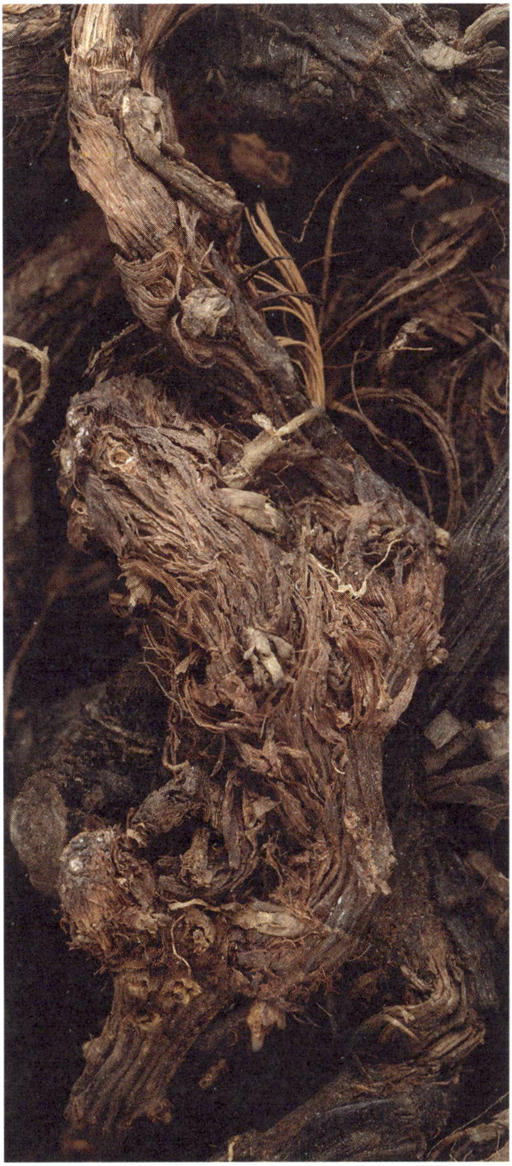

Main Qualities

It is one of the oldest oils. It has traditionally been a part of the incense used in many religious traditions.

Body/Skin

For millennia, it has been used as a healing agent for skin disturbances, a beauty aid for maintaining youthful skin, and a promoter of hair growth.

Mind/Emotions

As a relative of valerian, it is useful in treating insomnia and migraines.

Spiritual

It inspires devotion and promotes inner peace. It aids in finding spiritual and emotional balance and is essential to any spiritual blend.

Vetiver (Vetiveria zizanioides)

Family: Poaceae | Perfumery note: base | Aroma: woody, sweet, herbaceous

Vetiver oil, derived from vetiver grass found in tropical and subtropical regions, is known for its rich, earthy scent reminiscent of sandalwood or violets despite its narrow, odourless leaves. Commonly referred to as "khus" in India, this grass yields about 2.7 to 3.2 kg (six to seven lbs) of oil per tonne of crop annually, contributing to the global production of approximately 250 tonnes in 1987, primarily from Haiti and Indonesia. Vetiver roots, harvested after at least two years of growth and dried under the sun, are finely chopped, and the oil is extracted through methods like alcohol, acetone, benzene extraction, or distillation—the latter being favoured for therapeutic applications. With its warm, peppery, and woody aroma, the resulting dark brown oil plays a significant role in perfumery as a fixative. It is also featured in high-end soaps and aftershaves. Beyond its use in fragrances, vetiver has traditionally been used in India to flavour drinks and sweets and as a natural insect repellent. Its roots have been incorporated into mats, fans and window screens to cool homes and release its pleasant fragrance. At the same time, its oil has been used to safeguard textiles like cotton, furs and wool from moths, proving to be a more aromatic alternative to mothballs.

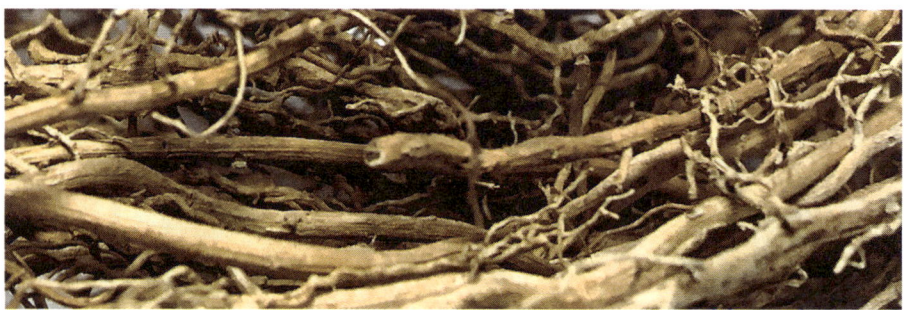

Main Qualities
Body/Skin

It is good for treating anorexia, stimulating the production of red blood cells, and beneficial for "aches and pains". It balances sebum production, treating both oily and dry skin and cooling the skin.

Mind/Emotions

Grounding and balancing make it a key ingredient in anti-anxiety blends. Relaxing when used as a mild sedative and useful for stress.

How To Use

Bath, compress, skincare, hair care, massage, perfume, room fragrance.

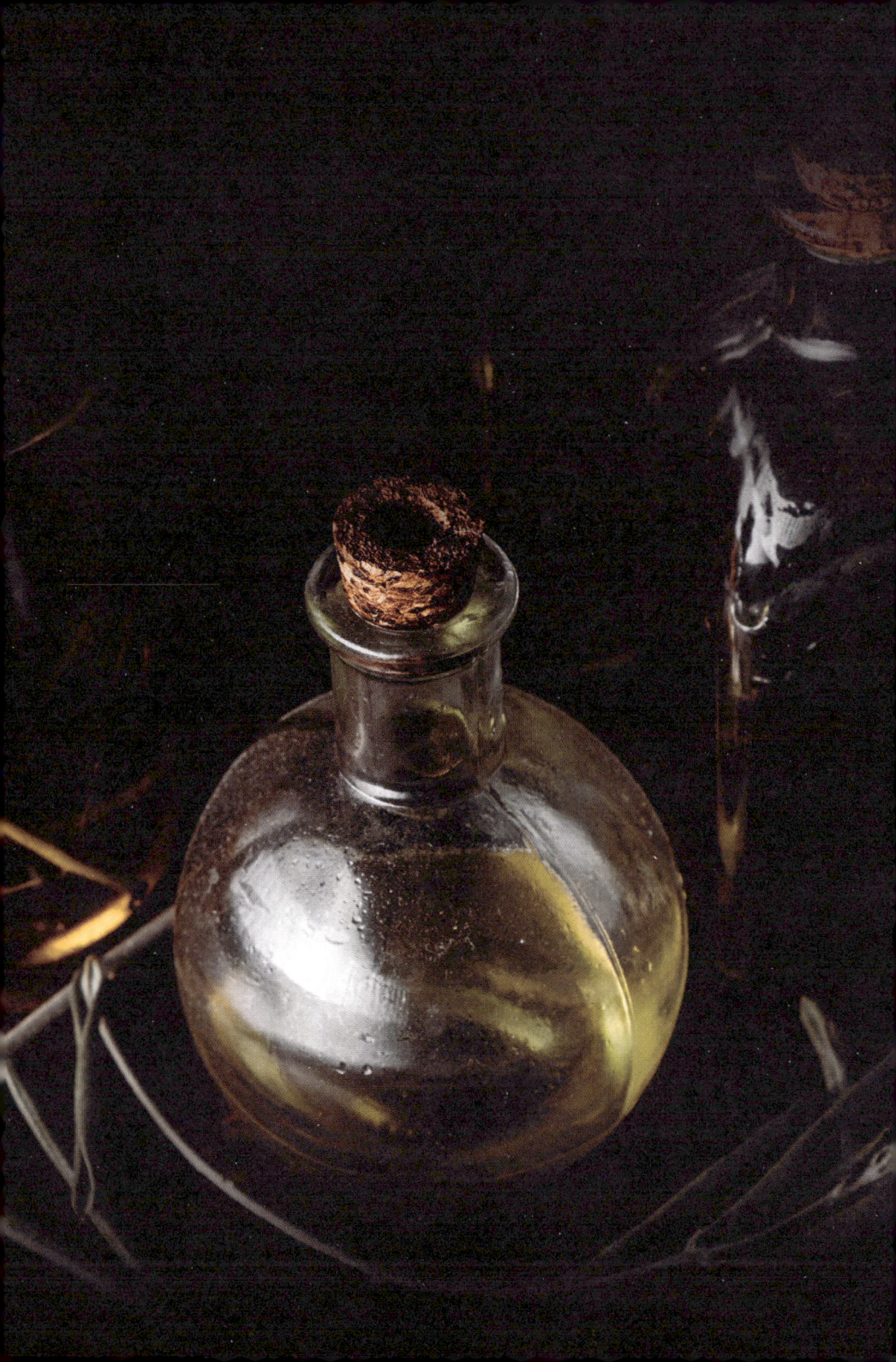

Chapter 6
Carrier or Base Oils

The base oils used in aromatherapy should be cold-pressed to retain their vitamin rich nature. Unlike essential oils, vegetable oils do not evaporate and serve as excellent natural bases for facials and body massage, showcasing their versatility and wide range of uses. Essential oils in their pure state are too concentrated to be used directly on the skin. Therefore, they are diluted in a carrier or base oil. Carrier oils are essential companions in the world of aromatherapy, serving as base oils used to dilute essential oils before they are applied to the skin. Derived from the fatty portions of plants, such as seeds, nuts, or kernels, carrier oils ensure that essential oils are safe for topical use, preventing skin irritation or sensitivity. Carrier oils are vital not only for safe application but also because they offer inherent beneficial properties. Rich in vitamins, minerals, and fatty acids, carrier oils nourish, moisturise, and protect the skin, enhancing the therapeutic effects of essential oils. By blending essential oils with carrier oils, aromatherapy practitioners can create customised, effective and luxurious treatments tailored to individual well-being.

Almond Sweet Oil:
Prunus Amygdalus

Contains: Glucosides, minerals, vitamins, and proteins

Uses: Good for all skin types. Helps relieve itching, soreness, dryness and inflammation.

Dilution: Can be used 100 per cent

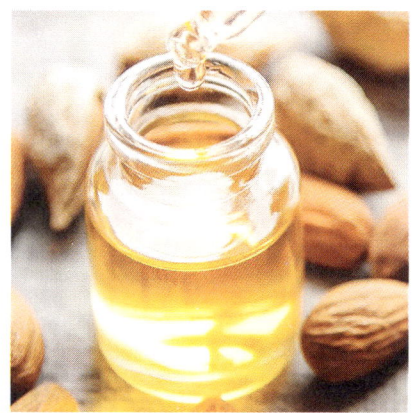

Apricot Kernel Oil:

Prunus Armeniaca

Contains: Vitamins and minerals

Uses: Good for all skin types, especially for prematurely aged, sensitive, inflamed, and dry.

Dilution: Can be used 100 per cent

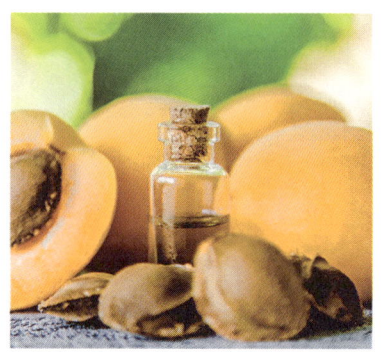

Avocado Oil:

Persea Americana

Contains: Vitamins, proteins, lecithin, and fatty acids

Uses: Good for all skin types, especially dry and dehydrated or eczema.

Dilution: Use 10 per cent

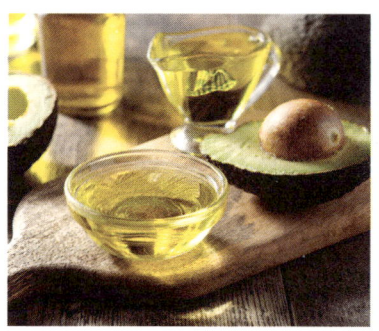

Castor Oil:

Ricinus Communis

Contains: Glyceride of ricinoleic, iso-ricinoleic, and lesser amounts of stearic, linoleic and dihydroxy stearic acids.

Uses: Helps dissolve cysts, growths, and warts, as well as soften corns and callouses. Prevents scars. Helpful for dry, chapped skin and conditions hair. Often recommended in addition with other oils for back pain. Avoid use during pregnancy.

Dilution: Use 10 per cent

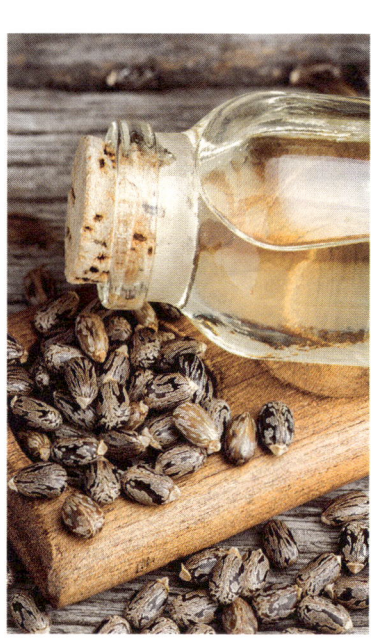

Carrier or Base Oils

Corn Oil:
Zea Mays

Contains: Proteins, vitamins, and minerals
Uses: soothing on all skin types.
Dilution: Can be used 100 per cent

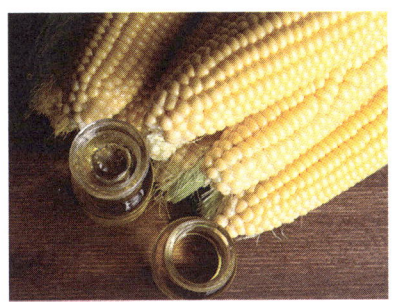

Evening Primrose Oil:
Oenothera Biennis

Contains: Gamma linolenic acid, vitamins, and minerals
Uses: Externally for psoriasis and eczema. Helps prevent prematurely aged skin and aids wound healing and any sort of dermatitis.
Dilution: Use 10 per cent

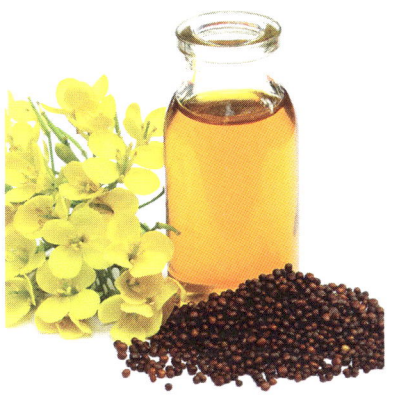

Grapeseed Oil:
Vitis Vinifera

Contains: Vitamins, minerals, proteins, and linoleic acid. Cholesterol free
Uses: For all skin types, odourless, penetrating. Very light oil. Slightly astrigent tightens and tones the skin. Does not aggravate acne.
Dilution: Can be used 100 per cent

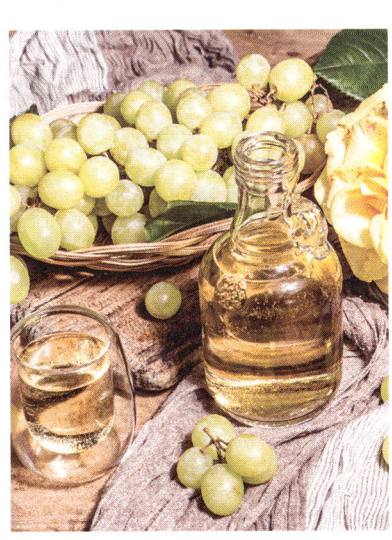

Hazelnut Oil:
Corylus Avellana

Contains: Vitamins, minerals, proteins, oleic acid, and linoleic acid
Uses: Slightly astringent, toning, fast absorption. Useful as a base for oily, combination skin and acne. Tones and tightens skin and maintains firmness and elasticity. Encourages cell regeneration and stimulates circulation.
Dilution: Can be used 100 per cent.

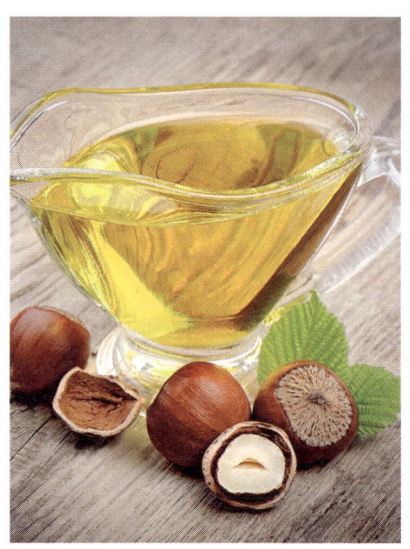

Jojoba Oil:
Simmondsia Chinensis

Contains: Protein, minerals, plant wax, and myristic acid
Uses: Similar to sebum, it penetrates the skin rapidly. Healing for inflamed skin, psoriasis, eczema, or any sort of dermatitis. Can help control acne and oily skin or scalp since excess sebum dissolves in jojoba. Antioxidant and may help extend the life of other oils. Also used for hair care. Useful for all skin types. Myristic acid is anti-inflammatory, so this could be a good base oil for treating rheumatism and arthritis.
Dilution: Use at 10 per cent or full strength.

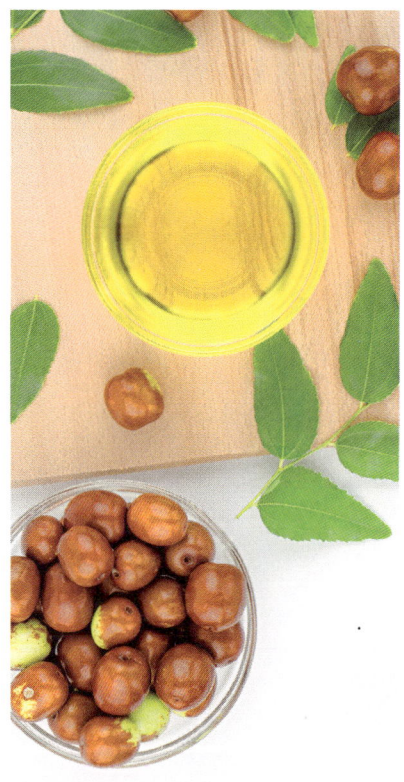

Carrier or Base Oils

Olive Oil:
Olea Europea

Contains: Proteins, minerals, vitamins
Uses: Rheumatic conditions, soothing, nail and hair care. Helpful acne skin, bruises and sprains. Strong odour makes it more useful with strongly scented essential oils.
Dilution: Use 10 per cent to 50 per cent Traditionally used to produce macerated oils.

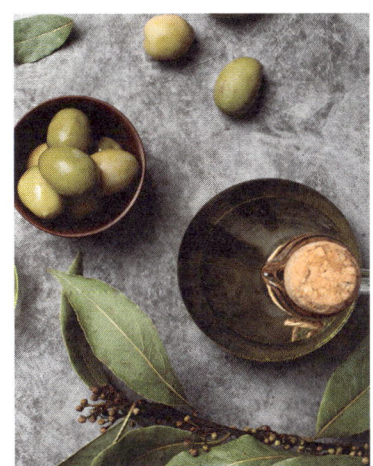

Sesame Oil (Til):
Sesamum Indicum

Contains: Vitamins especially vitamin E, minerals, proteins, lecithin, and amino acids
Uses: Psoriasis, rheumatism, arthritis, softening all skin types.
Dilution: Use 10 per cent to 100 per cent

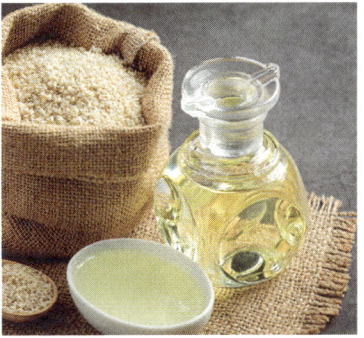

Sunflower Oil:
Helianthus Annuus

Contains: Vitamins A, B, D, E, minerals, lecithin, inulin, high in unsaturated fatty acids.
Uses: Suitable for all skin types, used to treat leg ulcers and skin diseases, bruises, diaper rash. Easily absorbed. Light textured.
Dilution: Can be used 100 per cent

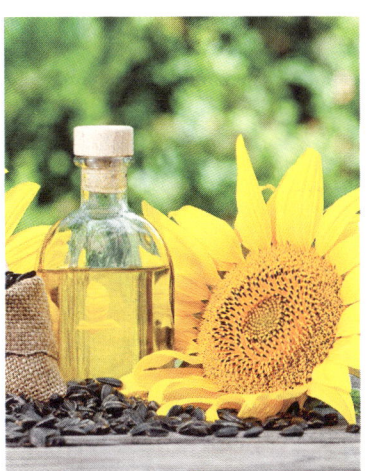

Carrier or Base Oils

Wheatgerm Oil:
Triticum Vulgare

Contains: Protein, minerals, and vitamins E, A, and D

Uses: Heals dry, cracked skin, eczema, psoriasis, prematurely aged skin, and stretch marks.

Note: Wheatgerm oil is often recommended as an addition to other oils to increase stability and shelf life. However, it can be dangerous for a person with severe wheat or gluten allergies.

Dilution: Use 10 per cent

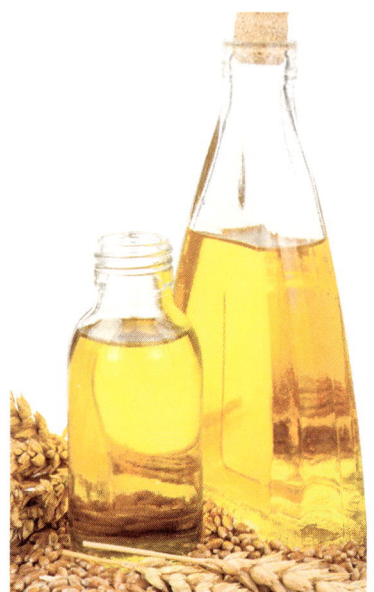

MACERATED (Infused) OILS

Macerated, or infused, oils are created by soaking plant materials in a carrier oil. This process allows the beneficial compounds from the plants to infuse into the oil, creating a rich blend that carries the therapeutic properties of both the plant and the carrier oil.

Carrot Oil:
Daucus Carota

Contains: Vitamins (B, C, D, E), minerals, beta carotene, provitamin A, and EFA's

Uses: For premature ageing, itching, burns, dryness, psoriasis and eczema; rejuvenating, reduces scarring.

Dilution: Use 10 per cent

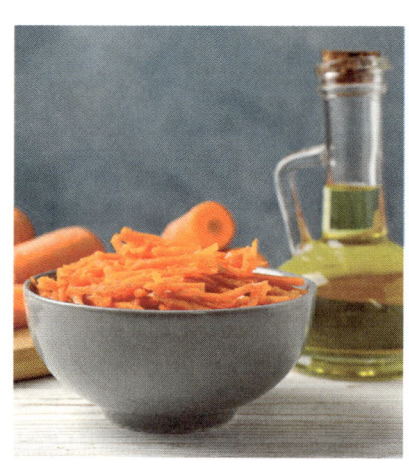

Carrier or Base Oils

Calendula Oil:
Calendula Officinalis

Contains: Salicylic acid, carotenoids, and phytosterols

Uses: Reduces swelling, aids wound and burn healing, and is helpful for acne, impetigo, and eczema. Antiseptic and regenerating. Some authorities and herbalists use full strength. Useful for bed sores, broken veins, bruises, inflamed gums, and varicose veins. Effective on rashes, dry, chapped or cracked skin. Wonderful in a blend for diaper rash. Especially useful for dry eczema.

Dilution: Use 10 per cent to 50 per cent.

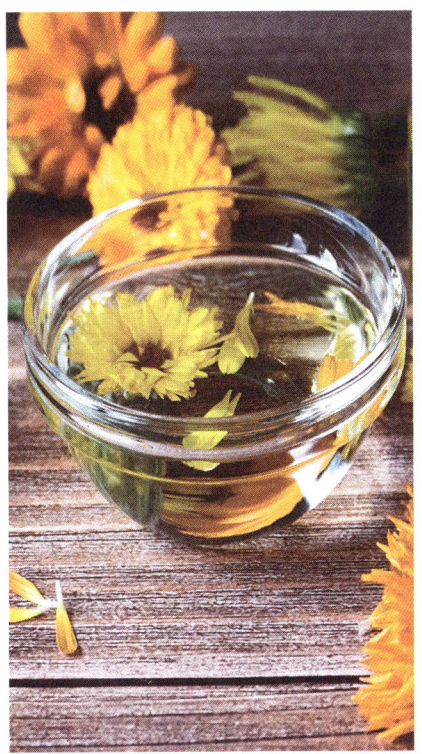

St John's Wort:
Hypericum Perforatum

Infused oil should have a characteristic red colour.

Uses: Anti-inflammatory, particularly soothing to inflamed nerves, helpful for cases of neuralgia, sciatica, and fibrositis. Effective on sprains, burns, and bruises. Blending with calendula oils heightens effectiveness.

Dilution: Use 10 per cent

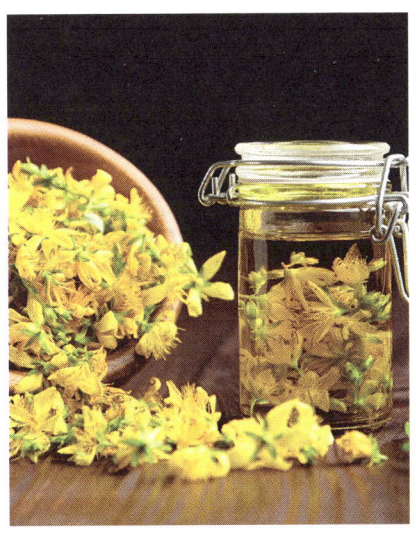

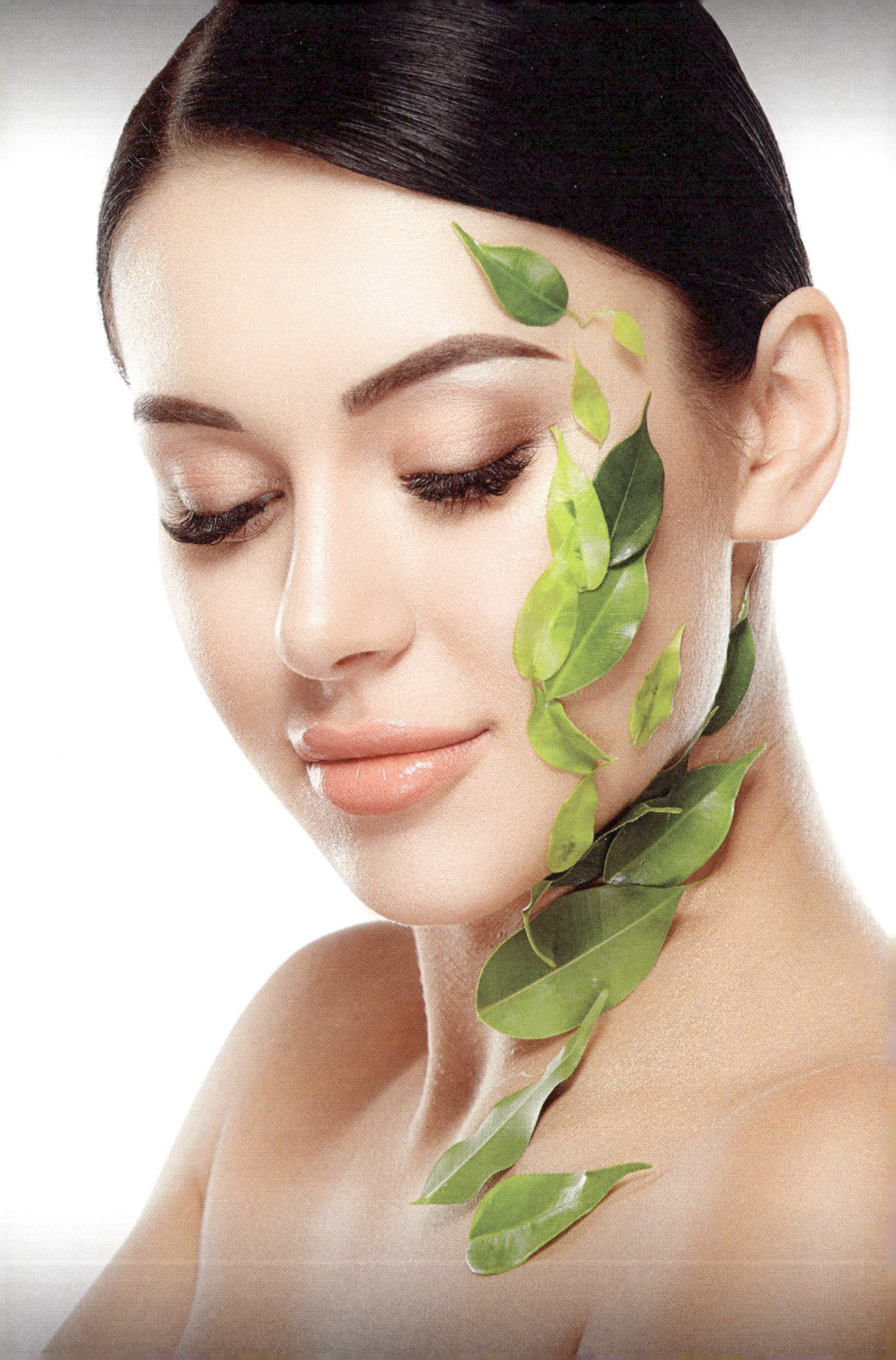

Chapter 7
Aromatherapy and Skincare

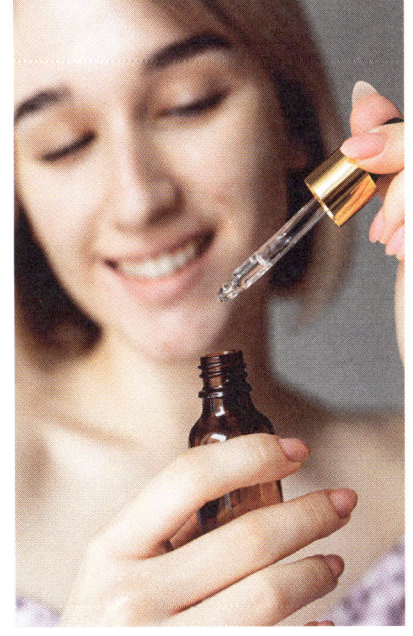

Essential oils in skincare have become increasingly popular as more people seek natural and holistic approaches to health and beauty. Essential oils offer powerful properties that, when harnessed in skincare routines, enhance the health and appearance of the skin, making them a valuable addition to any beauty regimen.

Benefits of Essential Oils in Skincare

Essential oils offer various benefits for the skin depending on their unique properties.

Antimicrobial and Antiseptic:

Highly effective in combating acne and preventing infections. They help cleanse the skin by eliminating bacteria, fungi and other pathogens that can cause skin issues. Promotes a clearer complexion by reducing the occurrence of breakouts.

Anti-Inflammatory:

Soothes and calms irritated skin. Beneficial for conditions such as eczema, rosacea, and psoriasis. Reduces redness, swelling, and discomfort, contributing to an even and calm skin tone and alleviating symptoms of inflammation and irritation.

Aromatherapy and Skincare

Antioxidant Protection:

Protects the skin from free radicals and environmental damage. Helps prevent premature aging, fine lines and wrinkles by neutralizing harmful molecules that can damage skin cells. Maintains a youthful and vibrant complexion.

Hydration and Moisturisation:

Locks in moisture and improves the skin's texture and elasticity. Penetrates deeply into the skin, providing long-lasting hydration and preventing dryness. Enhances the skin's natural barrier, keeping it soft, supple and nourished.

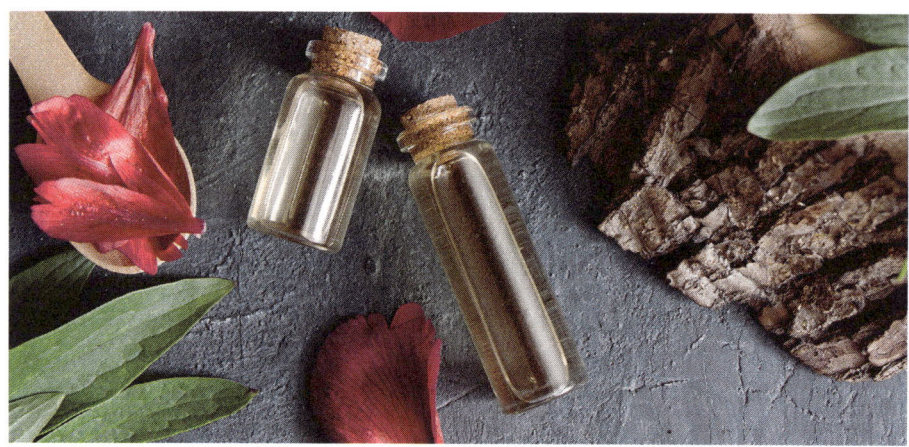

Skin Regeneration and Healing:

Promotes cell regeneration and healing to reduce the appearance of scars, fine lines and wrinkles. Stimulates the skin's natural repair processes, encouraging the growth of new healthy cells. Helps fade existing blemishes and improve overall skin tone and texture.

Incorporating Essential Oils into Skincare

To incorporate essential oils into your skincare routine, it's important to understand the correct usage and application methods:

1. Dilution:

Essential oils are highly concentrated and should be diluted with carrier oils like jojoba, almond or coconut oil to avoid skin irritation.

2. Patch Testing:

Before using a new essential oil, perform a patch test to ensure you do not have an adverse reaction.

3. Custom Blends:

Create custom blends tailored to your skin's needs. For example, a blend of tea tree and lavender oils can be effective for acne-prone skin, while a mix of frankincense and rose oil can benefit mature skin.

4. Application Methods:

Essential oils can be added to facial cleansers, toners, serums and moisturizers. They can also be used in facial steams, masks and baths for a more immersive experience.

Aromatherapy and essential oils offer a natural and effective way to enhance skincare routines, providing numerous benefits for various skin types and conditions. Understanding the properties and correct usage of these potent plant extracts can help you harness their full potential to achieve healthy and radiant skin. Whether you are looking to address specific skin concerns or wish to indulge in a luxurious and aromatic skincare experience, essential oils provide a versatile and holistic approach to skin health and beauty.

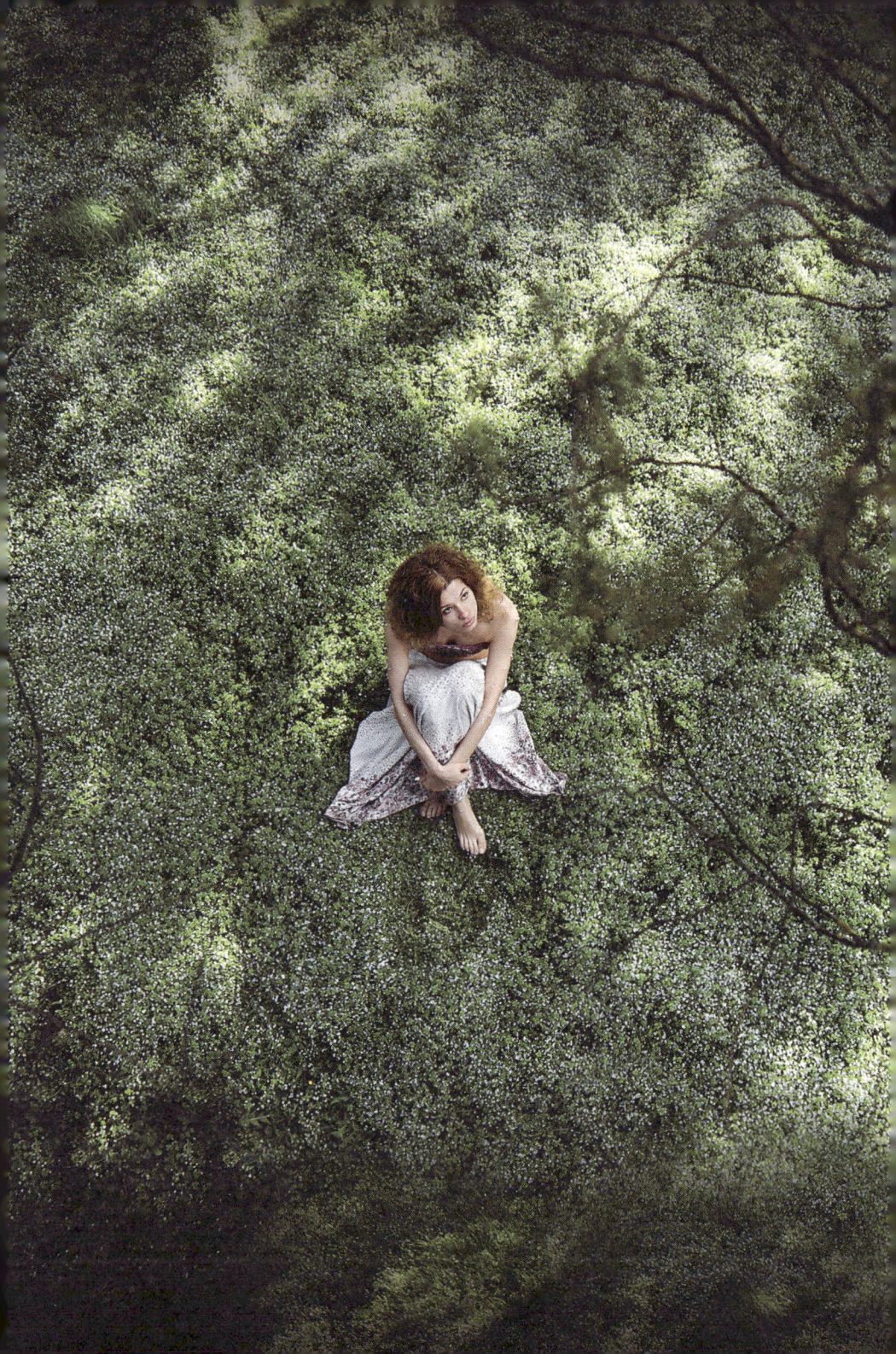

Chapter 8
Aromatherapy and Emotions

How Do Emotions Affect Health?

Emotions, whether positive or negative, wield a significant influence on our health. Positive emotions can bolster our health, while negative ones can inflict damage on our cells and overall well-being. Many of us unknowingly subject our health to the detrimental effects of negative emotions like anger, sadness, jealousy, guilt, resentment or disapproval. Recognizing these habitual emotions is a crucial first step towards enhancing our health and emotional well-being. By acknowledging these patterns, we can make changes that foster better emotional and physical health.

It's not always feasible to act on our emotions as they surface, so finding healthy ways to manage them without suppressing them is crucial. This necessitates finding constructive outlets for emotional relief. If emotions are bottled up or suppressed for an extended period without support, they can eventually harm our health. It's vital to address and process our emotions to sustain overall well-being.

While people can often manage their emotional responses, grief often presents a unique and complex challenge. Grief is a multifaceted emotional experience that unfolds without control over the event, involving stages such as disbelief, shock, denial, anger and acceptance. These stages underscore the need to traverse through grief with care to achieve emotional healing and uphold health. Touch is a fundamental human need that significantly

Aromatherapy and Emotions

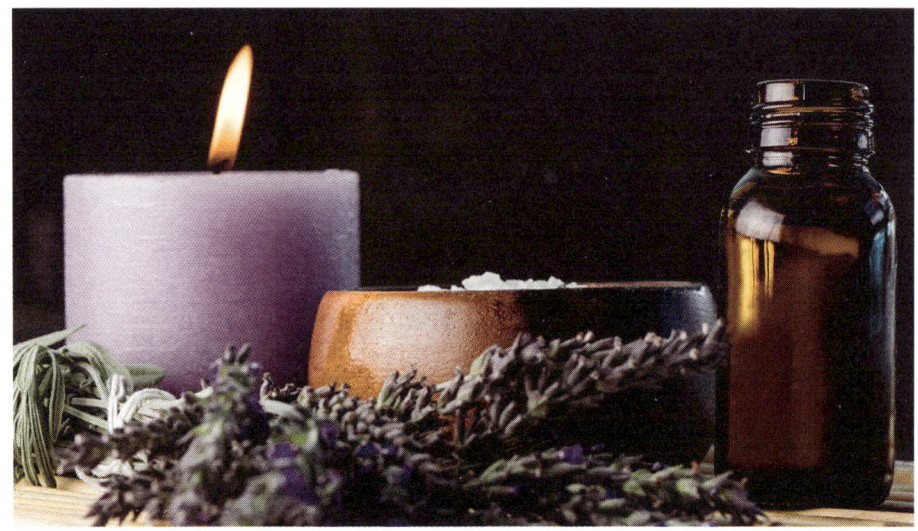

contributes to good health and soothing turbulent emotions. Our thoughts prompt us to reach out and the act of touching reflects those thoughts. Touch can also communicate emotions that are hard to put into words. Holding someone's hands or giving them a hug can often express our feelings more effectively than words, especially when comforting someone who is grieving.

Another important emotion is self-love, which doesn't mean thinking you're better or more important than others. It's about accepting yourself as you are, acknowledging any false beliefs you may hold and most importantly, having the ability to change things about yourself that you don't like or that undermine your confidence. Each positive change helps you love yourself a little more, empowering you and boosting your confidence. Forgiving is not always easy, but is it worth letting the rest of your life be ruined by something that happened in the past and only affects you, not the person responsible?

Forgiveness frees you from resentment, allowing you to start living positively and loving yourself and others, even those whose actions initially hurt you. You can stop feeling guilty, stop criticising yourself, forgive yourself and watch life

Aromatherapy and Emotions

begin to work in your favour. It's crucial to accept that what happened is in the past and cannot be changed. Blaming and criticizing those responsible only breeds unhappiness and resentment without any solution.

Aromas and Emotions

Aromas have a magical way of stirring emotions and memories, often intertwining the two. The sense of smell is deeply connected to our emotions, allowing scents to touch our hearts almost instantly. Essential oils embody this enchanting quality, holding powerful and mysterious energies that can evoke love, compassion and empathy. They act like messengers, carrying information and bridging different realms of experience. Through essential oils, we can connect with nature's wisdom, the universe's energy and the love within our hearts. Fragrances have the power to change our moods. We choose our thoughts—positive and uplifting or negative and harmful. What we think and believe tends to manifest in our lives. Just as the saying goes, We are what we eat, it's equally true that 'We are what we think.' The energy of essential oils interacts with our spiritual frequencies with their vibrational notes and creates harmony and peace. Essential oils possess a unique power to influence our entire being. They can heal wounds, relax the mind and uplift the soul. Their transformative power is unparalleled: they are adaptable, multifaceted, profoundly deep, light and subtle. If molecules could be angels, essential oils would be among them, bringing positive energy and transformation wherever they go.

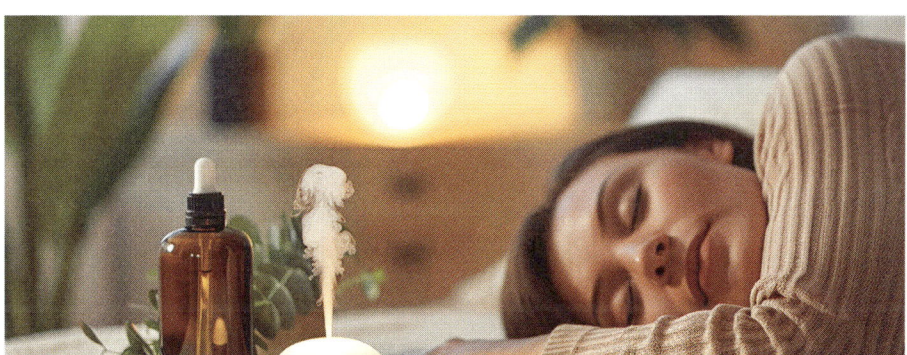

Aromatherapy and Emotions

For aromatherapy to be most effective, it should be part of a holistic lifestyle change:

- Eat wisely, give up smoking and consume alcohol and coffee in moderation.
- Engage in regular exercise even if it is just half an hour a day.
- Mix it up if you dislike routines.
- Take a walk, clean the kitchen or go for a swim.
- Recognize when you're tired and take a break. Pushing yourself increases stress.
- Enjoy a warm bath with essential oils and a soothing drink before bed.
- Make a list of important tasks and tackle them one at a time.
- Delegate tasks whenever possible to reduce stress.
- Be realistic about perfection and set attainable goals.

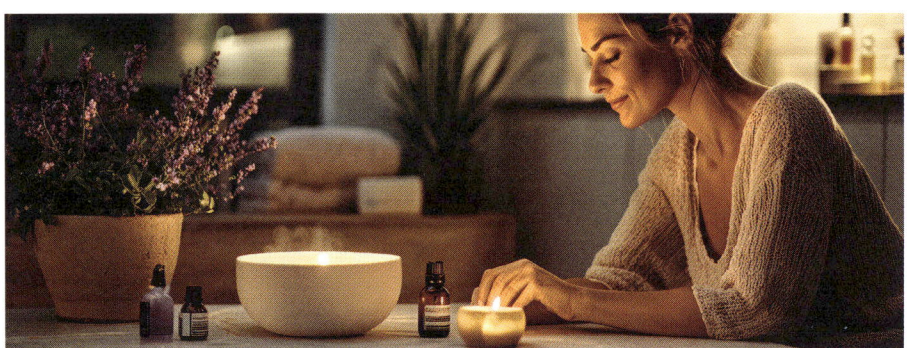

Grief | Distress | Deep Sorrow | Hurt | Anguish | Dejection | Despair | Hopelessness | Sadness

Grief is an emotion that, sooner or later, needs to be expressed and resolved. Talking about your grief with a close friend or allowing yourself to cry openly can provide some relief. Without these forms of emotional release, the weight of grief can linger much longer and be harder to manage.

Essential Oils that Help

Frankincense eases the mental pain of grief, especially in its early stages, by energising the nervous system and soothing distress. Its healing and antidepressant properties help both mental and physical wounds, while its calming effect promotes tranquillity and slows breathing, reducing future fears.

Marjoram balances and relaxes the nerves, alleviating grief-related pain and nervous depression. It also calms worries, agitation and loneliness.

Lavender soothes the nervous system, heals emotional wounds from bereavement and helps with depression.

Cypress supports emotional resilience and relaxation during the ups and downs of grief. It reduces irritability and remorse while instilling optimism.

Melissa provides instant calm for shock, helps with restlessness, anxiety, anger, and restores mental clarity.

Neroli helps with emotional shock, promotes sleep and alleviates deep emotional pain.

Rose uplifts the spirit, brings joy, and helps with mental fatigue and unresolved grief. It also cools anger and emotional stress while soothing fears about the future.

Anger | Irritability | Bitterness | Fury | Rage | Annoyance | Touchiness | Displeasure | Over-Sensitivity | Quick Temperedness | Impatience | Frustration | Dissatisfied | Disheartened

Anger can be one of the trickiest emotions to handle and is often repressed, which can negatively impact our lives. To address negative anger, we first need to acknowledge it. Frustration often triggers anger and while we're conditioned to see anger as a purely destructive force, it can also be a powerful catalyst for change when directed positively.

Aromatherapy and Emotions

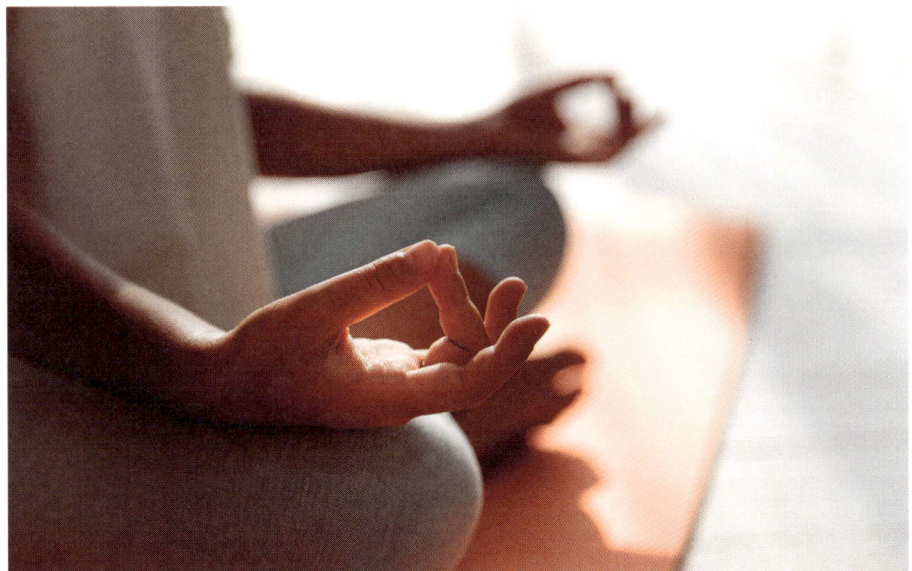

Properly managed, anger can be a constructive and assertive force; it only becomes negative when it's out of control. Unresolved anger can fester like an ulcer, leading to resentment, bitterness or even hatred and harming the soul and the body. This kind of anger can contribute to physical ailments like stomach ulcers and kidney stones. Essential oils can aid in releasing anger but positive thinking and faith in your ability to overcome challenges are also crucial. Practicing forgiveness is key to healing anger. Even if you don't feel it right away, repeatedly affirming 'I forgive them' can gradually shift your mindset towards genuine forgiveness. This approach, combined with relaxing essential oils, can significantly improve how you feel.

Essential Oils that Help

Roman Chamomile is a calming, sedative oil that soothes bursts of temper and helps address irritants that could evolve into deeper anger, like resentment. It also aids digestion and eases emotional upset linked to annoyance.

Bergamot's refreshing aroma supports forgiveness by releasing pent-up feelings and hidden anger. It promotes optimism and positive thinking.

Lavender encourages acceptance and can be particularly helpful when forgiveness feels challenging.

Lemon has an uplifting effect that helps shift your mood.

Geranium offers healing where anger has led to resentment or hatred. It soothes agitation, alleviates frustration and fosters acceptance and forgiveness.

Rosemary clears the mind, stimulates mental strength and helps protect against regrettable retaliation.

Fear | Apprehension | Alarm | Anxiety | Agitation | Panic | Terror

Fear often lies at the heart of anxiety. Depending on its intensity and duration, fear can be both painful and potentially harmful. It's important not to be ashamed of our fear but to acknowledge it as a natural part of who we are. Coping with fear in a healthy way is crucial for maintaining our well-being. Using essential oils proactively can help manage fear when facing new situations.

Essential Oils that Help

Basil Sweet is known for easing nervous disorders and is ideal for calming a heart troubled by strong emotions. It helps soothe an anxious heart, clears and strengthens the mind and promotes serenity. Basil Sweet also relaxes the body and alleviates fear induced nausea.

Melissa lowers blood pressure, calms the body and normalizes a rapid heartbeat by easing feelings of dread and apprehension.

Marjoram supports the nervous system, promotes restful sleep and relieves the tightness in the chest and sweating that fear can cause.

Aromatherapy and Emotions

Bergamot acts as a sedative for the nervous system, providing the courage to face challenging situations.

Lavender helps lower blood pressure, improves sleep, and boosts courage during moments of apprehension.

Jealousy | Envy | Unhappiness | Resentment | Annoyance | Displeasure | Dissatisfaction | Spite | Hatred | Grudge | Malice | Bitterness

Jealousy is often intertwined with anger and resentment, potentially escalating into intense fury and violence. Envy is less volatile and desire can be mostly innocent, yet both can also evolve into stronger emotions. One can experience the following as part of jealousy: an inability to share, unfulfilled ambition, dissatisfaction with what one has or an overly suspicious mind. These factors can lead to feelings of resentment and difficulty accepting and appreciating what we already have. Admitting jealousy or envy can be challenging, but acknowledging it is crucial because it is a highly destructive emotion. Jealousy not only harms ourselves but can also negatively affect others. Some individuals may isolate themselves from friends with qualities or achievements they covet, such as successful careers, harmonious relationships, or physical traits. Jealousy acts like a mental toxin, consuming and invading our being.

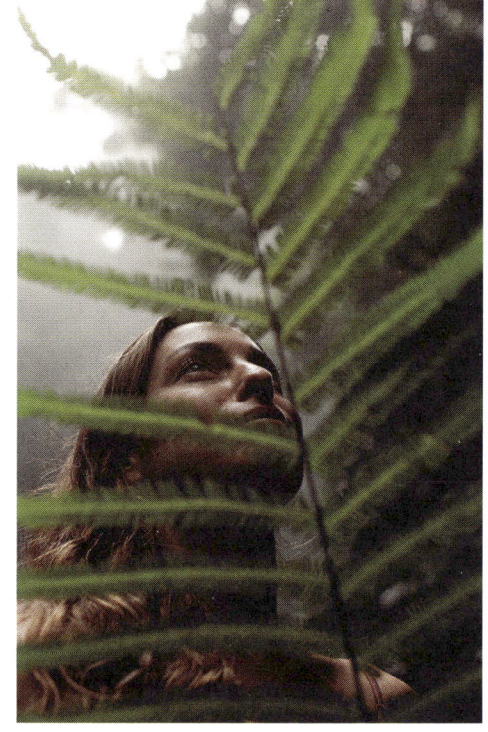

Essential Oils that Help

Juniper is known for its detoxifying properties and has the ability to dissolve stubborn, negative emotions and clear them from the mind.

Basil Sweet helps eliminate emotions that gnaw at us internally and can aid in healing stomach ulcers, suggesting its effectiveness in easing mild and troubling emotions. It strengthens the heart and mind, promoting clear thinking about how jealousy can negatively impact health.

Bergamot is refreshing and helps release anger. If jealousy or envy has become a persistent issue leading to depression, bergamot's neurotonic properties can uplift your spirits, while its sedative effects soothe and help release pent-up emotions.

Lemon assists in dissolving the negative, hostile feelings associated with jealousy, clearing away worthless emotions.

Guilt | Remorse | Regret | Fear of Disgrace | Shame

Guilt often stems from not valuing yourself, prioritizing family needs over your own emotions or feeling ashamed about overeating and weight issues. This type of guilt can be tied to shame over past mistakes and can create ongoing internal conflict. You might feel like you need to atone for enjoying yourself or believe you don't deserve affection from loved ones. This can lead to excessive apologising and helping others even when you're not willing or able. Positive thinking is key to overcoming guilt and essential oils can help ease these feelings, making them more manageable and shift your attitude towards life.

Essential Oils that Help

Lavender is an excellent choice for healing mental anguish and self-reproach.

Frankincense can uplift your spirits and energise you, relieving self-directed anger and easing feelings of guilt.

Aromatherapy and Emotions

Apathy | Lack of Feeling | Indifference | Lack of Enthusiasm | Lack of Energy | Boredom

Apathy often reflects a 'don't care' attitude and may be linked to feelings of inadequacy. Beneath this attitude, you might experience hopelessness, disappointment, boredom or even suppressed chronic anger. It tends to develop slowly, often resulting from a pattern of choosing the easy path.

Essential Oils that Help

Juniper helps cleanse and purify the mind, shaking off sluggish and inactive energy. It strengthens willpower and rekindles determination.

Ginger stimulates the senses and boosts spirits, addressing fatigue and revitalising drive and motivation.

Clary Sage is effective for managing mental fatigue, clearing the mind and removing toxins. It offers a mental and emotional uplift, restoring clarity and encouraging regeneration.

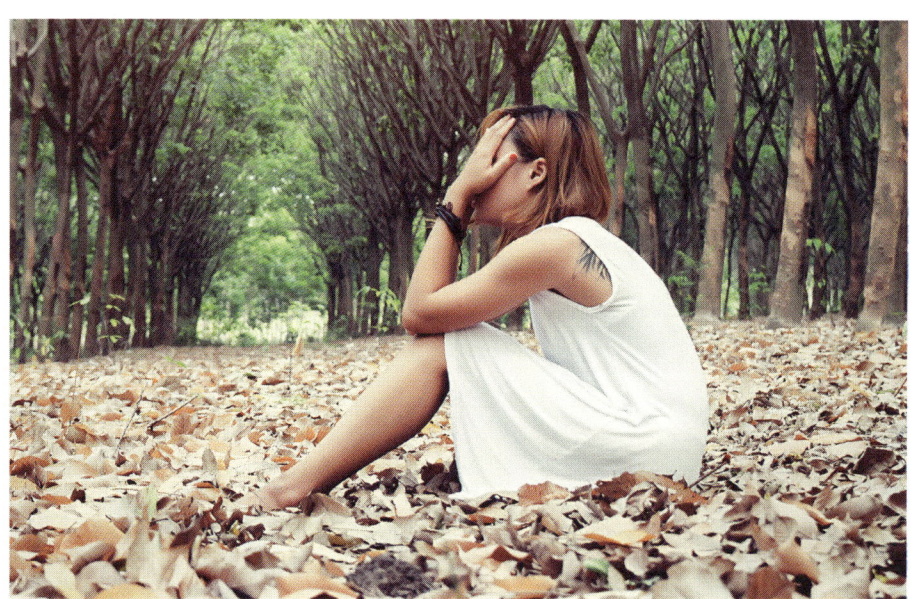

Aromatherapy and Emotions

Mood Swings | Gloomy | Sulky | Emotional | Excitable | Impatient | Irritable Sensitive

Positive moods can range from feeling vibrant and enthusiastic to relaxed and tired. Negative moods, on the other hand, can fluctuate from being antagonistic and worried to irritable and good-natured or from unhappy to happy, often showing inconsistency. For women, mood swings that alternate between irritability and cheerfulness or unhappiness and joy are often linked to the reproductive system and are commonly experienced before menstruation and during menopause. Several essential oils can help balance these emotional shifts.

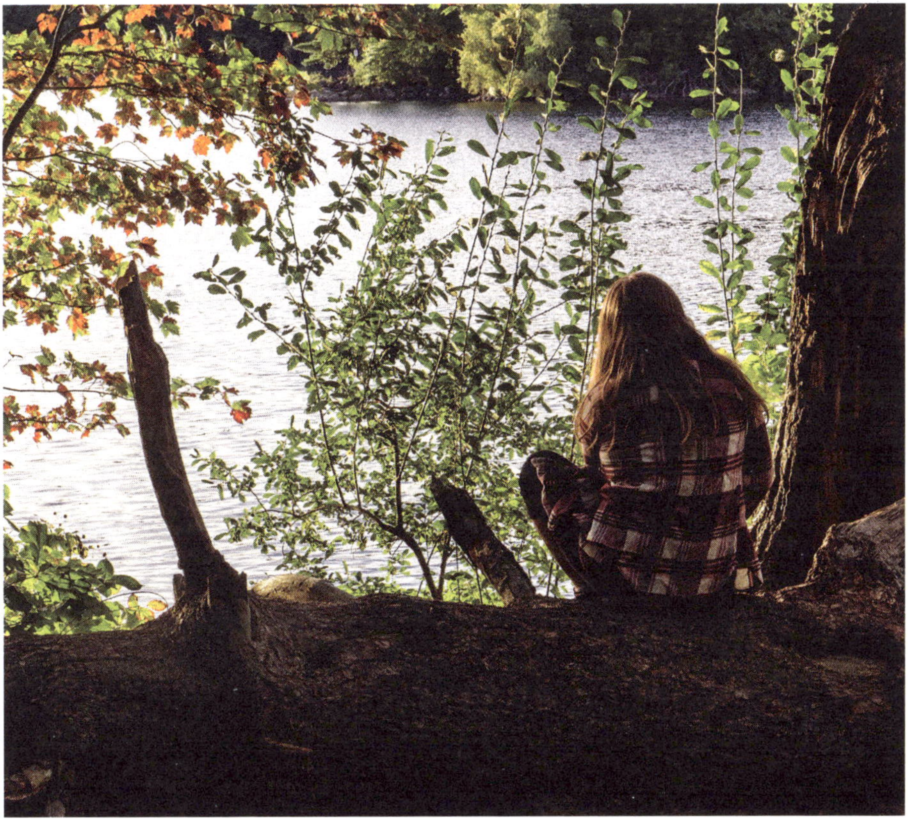

Aromatherapy and Emotions

Essential Oils that Help

Clary Sage is a classic choice for managing mood swings. It is known for its neurotonic properties, which help calm irritability and alleviate feelings of jealousy and envy. This makes it ideal for emotional confusion and fluctuating moods.

Geranium is effective in calming anxiety and lifting the heaviness of depression. It can also act as a sedative for agitation or irritation, helping to stabilize the mood.

Lavender is renowned for its calming effects and ability to strengthen the heart, making it an excellent choice for general moodiness. It helps balance emotional instability and regulate mood fluctuations.

Timidity | Shyness | Unworthiness | Underachievement | Lack of Confidence

These feelings can significantly impact your ability to reach your potential and enjoy life to the fullest. Timidity can stem from a fear of judgment or rejection, making it challenging to assert or engage in social situations, leading to missed opportunities and a sense of isolation.

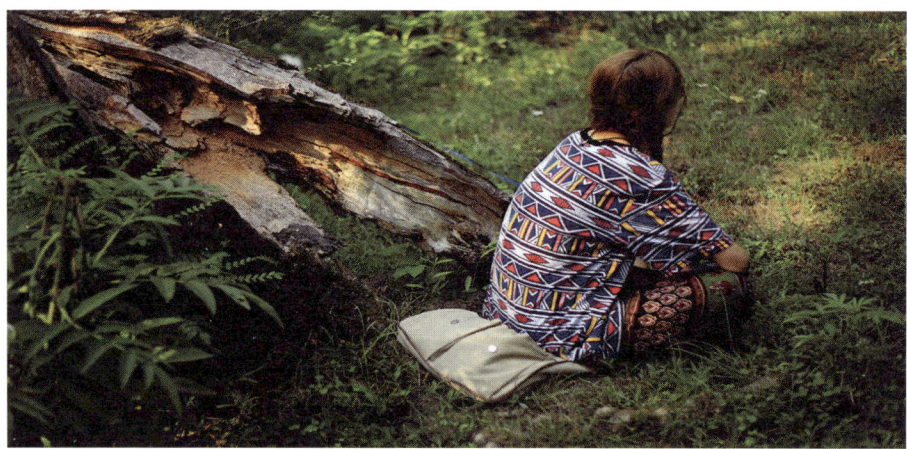

Aromatherapy and Emotions

A deep-seated feeling that you do not deserve success, love or respect; unworthiness can be rooted in past experiences, societal expectations, or internalized criticism. It can lead to self-sabotage when coupled with a lack of confidence and you might not accept positive experiences, believing you don't deserve them.

Essential Oils that Help

Fennel's stimulating and tonic qualities help revitalise your emotions, boosting your energy and drive.

Sweet Marjoram alleviates feelings of neglect, bringing warmth and reassurance that you are cared for.

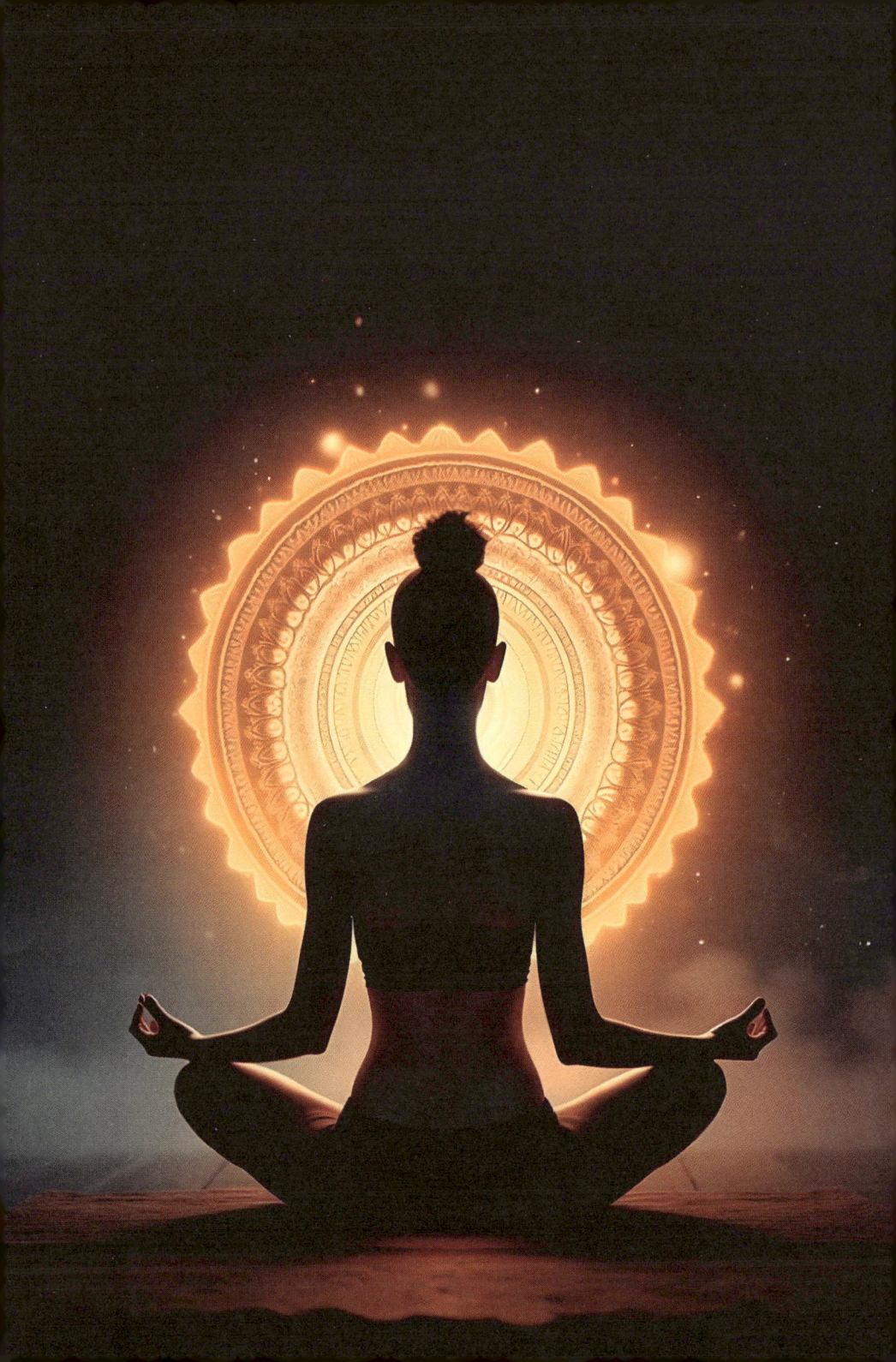

CHAPTER 9

Aromatherapy and Chakras

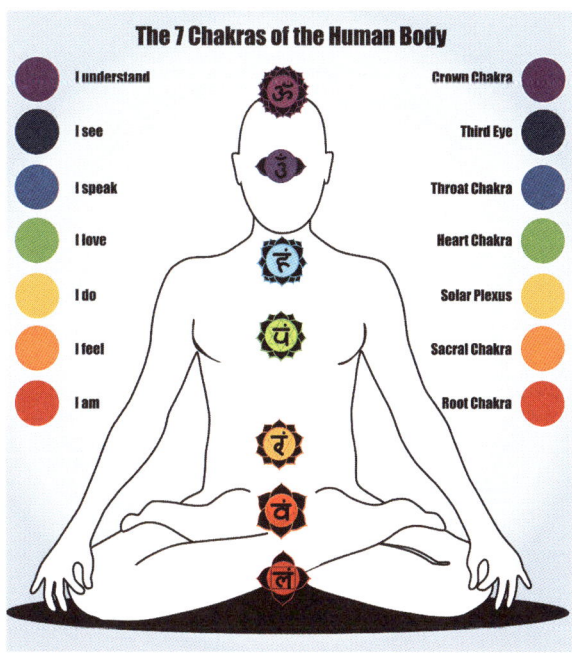

Aromatherapy offers a delightful and sensory-rich approach to wellness, intertwining the aromatic essences of the natural world with our personal health practices. It's particularly enchanting when combined with the concept of chakras, which means 'wheel', the vibrant, spinning energy centres that govern various physical, emotional and spiritual aspects of our lives. According to ancient traditions such as Ayurveda and yoga, maintaining balance among these chakras promotes a harmonious flow of energy throughout the body, improving overall well-being.

Each chakra, from the base of the spine to the crown of the head, corresponds to different life themes and body functions. Because chakras are centres of moving energy, they can become blocked or vibrate too much or too little, becoming overactive or underactive. When you experience a blocked, overactive or underactive chakra, your mental, spiritual and physical health can suffer. Aromatherapy can be a supportive tool in nurturing and balancing

Aromatherapy and Chakras

these energy centres by using specific essential oils known for their unique properties. This holistic approach enhances the body's subtle energy and appeals to our sense of smell, deeply influencing our mental and emotional states.

1. ROOT | MULADHARA
GROUNDING | I AM *safe, grounded, supported*
Location: base of spine
Colour: red

When your root chakra is balanced, you'll experience a profound sense of satisfaction and peace, particularly in crucial life areas such as finances, home and personal safety. A well-aligned root chakra fosters a warm connection to the earth, enhancing your everyday experiences. It forms a sturdy base for personal growth, providing a comforting sense of security and stability. Moreover, a balanced root chakra is beneficial for your physical health, contributing to your overall strength and well-being.

Overactive Root Chakra

- Resentment or anger towards others
- Greediness
- Difficulty accepting change
- Impatience
- Digestive issues
- Lower back or hip pain
- Procrastination
- Suicidal tendencies
- Insomnia

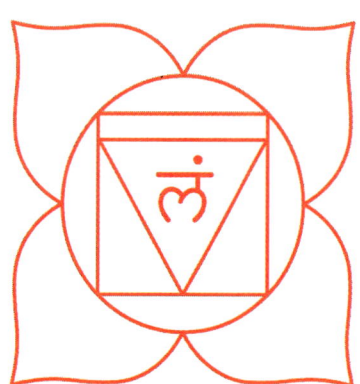

Underactive Root Chakra

Insecurity of feeling secure or lack of a sense of home

- Disorganized
- Lack of focus
- Feelings of nervousness, anxiety, or fear of abandonment
- Disassociation
- Difficulty finding financial security

When imbalanced, you feel

Anxiety, instability, lack of self-esteem and motivation, disconnected, cynicism

When balanced, you feel

Security, stability, grounding, enthusiasm, commitment

Diffuse or apply essential oils that have an earthy aroma and grounding effects. Apply oils to your feet, legs, and the base of the spine. Always mix with a base oil before application.

Vetivert | Can help you feel grounded and centred in yourself, as well as encourage emotional strength.

Patchouli | Provides feelings of relaxation and helps ease stress or anxiety.

Myrrh | Helps you relax and calm your nerves.

Frankincense | Gives you the ability to read environmental energy and help prevent reactivity.

2. SACRAL | SWADISHTANA
CREATIVITY | I FEEL *creative, confident, passion*
Location: lower abdomen
Colour: orange

When your sacral chakra is balanced, you can fully embrace and enjoy life's

Aromatherapy and Chakras

pleasures without going overboard. This chakra is your centre for experiencing emotions deeply and forming intimate connections. It fuels your creative fires and inspires you to pursue your passions with enthusiasm. A well-tuned sacral chakra enriches your relationships and enhances your ability to express yourself artistically and explore new ideas. It's essential for feeling a sense of wellness and zest in your daily life, helping you engage with the world in more meaningful and vibrant ways.

Overactive Sacral Chakra

- Overly emotional, moody or dramatic
- Strong emotions of anxiety or aggression
- Increased emotional attachment to others
- Lack of personal boundaries
- Addictions or gluttony
- Restlessness

Underactive Sacral Chakra

- Lack of creativity
- Greater insecurity
- Emotionally closed off from others
- Frigidity or lack of desire
- Fear or shame of intimacy
- Sluggishness

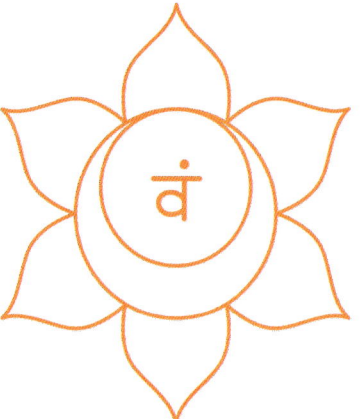

When imbalanced, you feel

Fear of intimacy, emotional and physical weakness, oversensitivity, lack of libido

When balanced, you feel

Vitality, creativity, joy, prosperity, passion, pleasure

Aromatherapy and Chakras

Diffuse or apply essential oils that have cleansing and balance effects. Apply oils to your lower abdomen, just beneath the navel. Always mix with a base oil before application.

Ylang Ylang | Helps reduce anxiety and boosts self-esteem.

Rose | Soothes and relaxes, bringing feelings of happiness and passion.

Sweet Orange | Activates the chakra and brings forth your sense of creativity and play.

Patchouli | Balances and grounds your emotions.

Tangerine | Relieves stress and tension, balances your emotions, and promotes feelings of joy.

Neroli | Helps balance an overactive sacral chakra, relieving anxiety and promoting well-being.

Jasmine | Balances hormones and helps with emotional balance and creativity.

3. SOLAR PLEXUS | MANIPURA
PURPOSE | *I DO confidence, focus, ambition, self-assertiveness*
Location: above the navel
Colour: yellow

When your solar plexus chakra is balanced, you feel a strong sense of self and a deep alignment with your true identity. This chakra relates to personal power and control over your thoughts, actions, and emotions. It fuels your self-discipline and drives you to accomplish your goals.

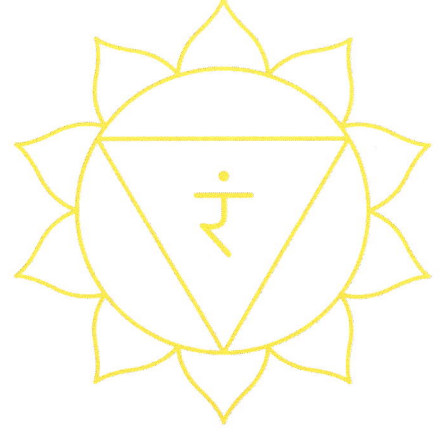

As the core of your confidence, a balanced solar plexus chakra enhances your self-esteem and empowers you to trust your abilities, helping you face life's challenges with a strong and confident spirit.

Overactive Solar Plexus

- A desire to be in control or micromanage others
- Feelings of anger or aggression
- Lack of compassion or empathy
- Digestive issues
- Perfectionism or being overly critical
- Jealousy, cruelty, greed

Underactive Solar Plexus

- Lack of confidence and low self-esteem
- Indecisiveness
- Greater timidness
- Seeking external approval and worrying about what others think
- Neediness

When imbalanced, you feel

Weakness, low self-esteem, inferiority, fear of rejection, indecisiveness, jealousy, hatred, intolerance

When balanced, you feel

Energy, confidence, drive, abundance

Diffuse or apply essential oils that promote confidence, motivation, and courage. Apply the oils to your abdomen a few inches above the navel in the hollow area between the ribs. Always mix with a base oil before application.

Sandalwood | Helps you align with your most authentic self.

Aromatherapy and Chakras

Myrrh | Soothing for nerves and helps relax.

Cedarwood | Reduces stress and anxiety and increases your energy.

Lemongrass | Uplifts and invigorates, bringing hope and enthusiasm.

Lavender | Reduces anxiety and stress.

Helichrysum | Brings out confidence and hidden personal power.

Juniper | Improves circulation and releases stuck energy.

4. HEART | ANAHATA
LOVE | *I LOVE peace, compassion*
Location: centre of chest
Colour: green

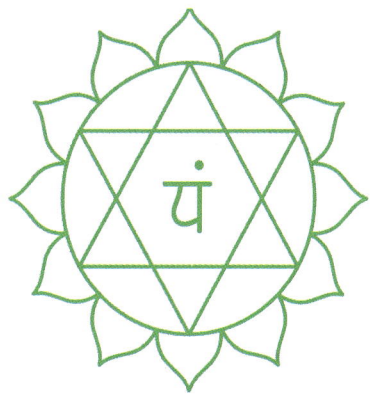

When your heart chakra is balanced, you will find it easier to connect deeply with others, whether in family, friendships or romantic relationships. This chakra empowers you to embrace compassion, helping you understand and feel what others are experiencing. With a balanced heart chakra, you can love unconditionally and are more open to letting go of past hurts and forgiving those who have wronged you. It enables you to move past old wounds and welcome new experiences and relationships with open arms. Additionally, a healthy heart chakra means you can love yourself just as freely as you do others, creating a life filled with genuine connections and heartfelt moments.

Overactive Heart Chakra

- Lack of control over emotions
- Clingy or lack of personal boundaries
- Saying 'yes' to everything, even if it hurts you

- Lack of sense of self in relationships
- Feelings of jealousy or superiority

Underactive Heart Chakra

- Isolation or distance in relationships
- Cold demeanour or lack of empathy towards others
- Unforgiving and grudgeful
- Overly critical of others and yourself
- Not willing to open up to others

When imbalanced, you feel

Loneliness, lack of self-love, insecurity, suppressed higher emotions

When balanced, you feel

Love, empathy, compassion, acceptance, openness, fulfilment, joy

Diffuse or apply essential oils that are uplifting and promote feelings of love, positivity, and joy. Apply oils to your chest area. Always mix with a base oil before application.

Rose | Brings forth feelings of love.

Pine | Relieves emotional pain and helps you move forward.

Jasmine | Promotes a sense of calmness and balance in life.

Ylang Ylang | Eases anxiety and boosts compassion.

Geranium | Assists in opening up to self-love and self-healing.

5. THROAT | VISUDDHA
EXPRESSION | I SPEAK *communication, self-expression*
Location: base of neck - throat
Colour: blue

Aromatherapy and Chakras

When your throat chakra is balanced, you will feel empowered to be your authentic self and express your thoughts and feelings openly. This chakra motivates you to speak your truth and stand firm in your beliefs. As the centre of communication, a balanced throat chakra enhances your ability to share 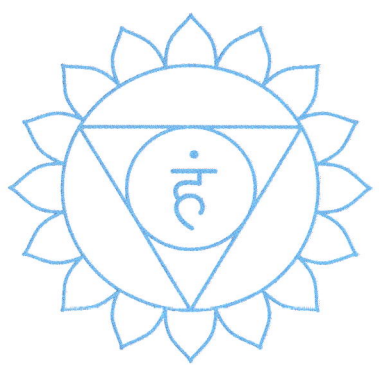 and articulate ideas. It also boosts your creativity and inspiration. It's all about expressing yourself clearly and confidently, whether it's through words, art or other creative outlets.

Overactive Throat Chakra

- Inability to listen to others
- Overly critical
- Overly talkative and interruptive
- Feeling like you aren't heard by others
- Throat pain or discomfort

Underactive Throat Chakra

- Shutting down as a result of not being heard
- Introverted, shy or timid
- Difficulty speaking up
- Unable to express yourself or your needs

When imbalanced, you feel

Shyness, weak voice, underconfident, lack of creativity and expression

When balanced, you feel

Confidence, creativity, self-expression and effective communication

Aromatherapy and Chakras

Diffuse or apply essential oils that encourage creativity and clarity. Apply oil to your throat area and around the ears. Always mix with a base oil before application.

Chamomile | Calms and relaxes, helping you to speak your inner truth.
Peppermint | Regenerates energy within the body and clears blockages.
Frankincense | Gives you the clarity to respond with grace and encourages clear, effective speech.
Spearmint | Invigorates and brings forth fresh ideas.

6. THIRD EYE | AJNA

INTUITION | I SEE *intuition, clarity, imagination, understanding*
Location: between the eyebrows
Colour: indigo

When your third eye chakra is balanced, it opens your mind to deeper understanding and broader knowledge.

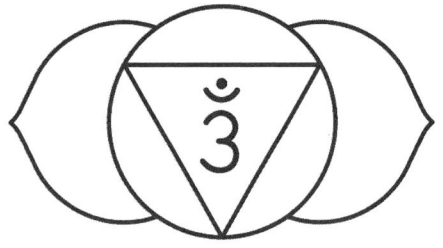

This chakra is vital to how you perceive the world, enhancing your intuition and encouraging profound inner reflection. With a balanced third eye chakra, you are more open to exploring your thoughts and feelings, gaining insights that were previously out of reach. It acts as a bridge between your inner mind and the external world, helping you to integrate your mental insights with your physical experiences. This connection fosters a well-rounded perspective, allowing you to see and understand more than ever before.

Overactive Third Eye Chakra

- Lacking good judgement

- Inability to focus
- Feeling mentally overwhelmed
- Overanalyzing
- Mental fog

Underactive Third Eye Chakra

- Rigid, inflexible thinking
- Not open to new ideas
- Fearful of the future
- Lack of intuition
- Inability to self-reflect

When imbalanced, you feel

Lack of imagination, poor judgement, fearfulness, inattentiveness

When balanced, you feel

Clear thinking, intuition, focus, mental strength, insight, consciousness

Diffuse or apply essential oils that encourage balance and clarity of mind. Apply oils between the eyes and along the forehead. Always mix with a base oil before application.

Lemon | Encourages deep thought processes and creative spark, uplifting.

Sandalwood | Soothes and imparts feelings of happiness.

Rosemary | Fresh and invigorating, can increase mental function.

Cedarwood | Helps you connect to nature and clears confusion and indecisiveness.

Clary Sage | Clears negative emotions and toxic energy from your aura and space.

7. CROWN | SAHASRARA
BLISS | I KNOW *intuition, wisdom, spiritual growth*
Location: top of the head - crown area
Colour: violet

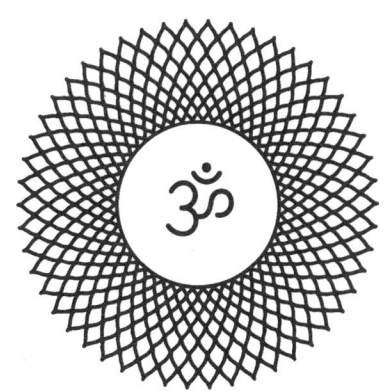

When your crown chakra is balanced, you can appreciate the beauty and divine role of everything around you. This chakra connects you with the universe, fostering a sense of unity with everyone and everything.

A well-aligned crown chakra lifts your consciousness, enhancing your clarity and understanding of the physical and cosmic realms. With a balanced crown chakra, you'll find yourself experiencing deeper peace, serenity, and joy, feeling more connected and harmonious with the world.

Overactive Crown Chakra

- Lack of empathy
- Feelings of indifference and superiority
- Disconnection between your body and the earth
- Addiction to spirituality, trying to feel connected
- Difficulty controlling emotions

Underactive Crown Chakra

- Closed off to spirituality
- Lack of personal direction

- Unable to keep goals
- Greed and materialism
- Mental fog

When imbalanced, you feel

Depression, forgetfulness, lack of purpose, materialism, sense of fear

When balanced, you feel

Faith, universal love, open-mindedness, oneness with universe

Diffuse or apply essential oils that uplift your spirits and inspire enlightenment. Apply oils to the crown of your head. Always mix with a base oil before application.

Rose | Soothes and relaxes, enhancing spiritual connection.

Lavender | Calming and soothing, promoting sleep that helps balance the chakra.

Myrrh | Relaxing and promoting spiritual awareness.

Neroli | Helps you stay focused on the present moment, not on the past or the future.

Sandalwood | Assists with meditation and bringing you to a higher frequency.

Jasmine | Boosts mood, instils feeling of tranquillity.

Lotus | Balances and activates the chakra, promoting a sense of spiritual well-being and deepens meditation practices.

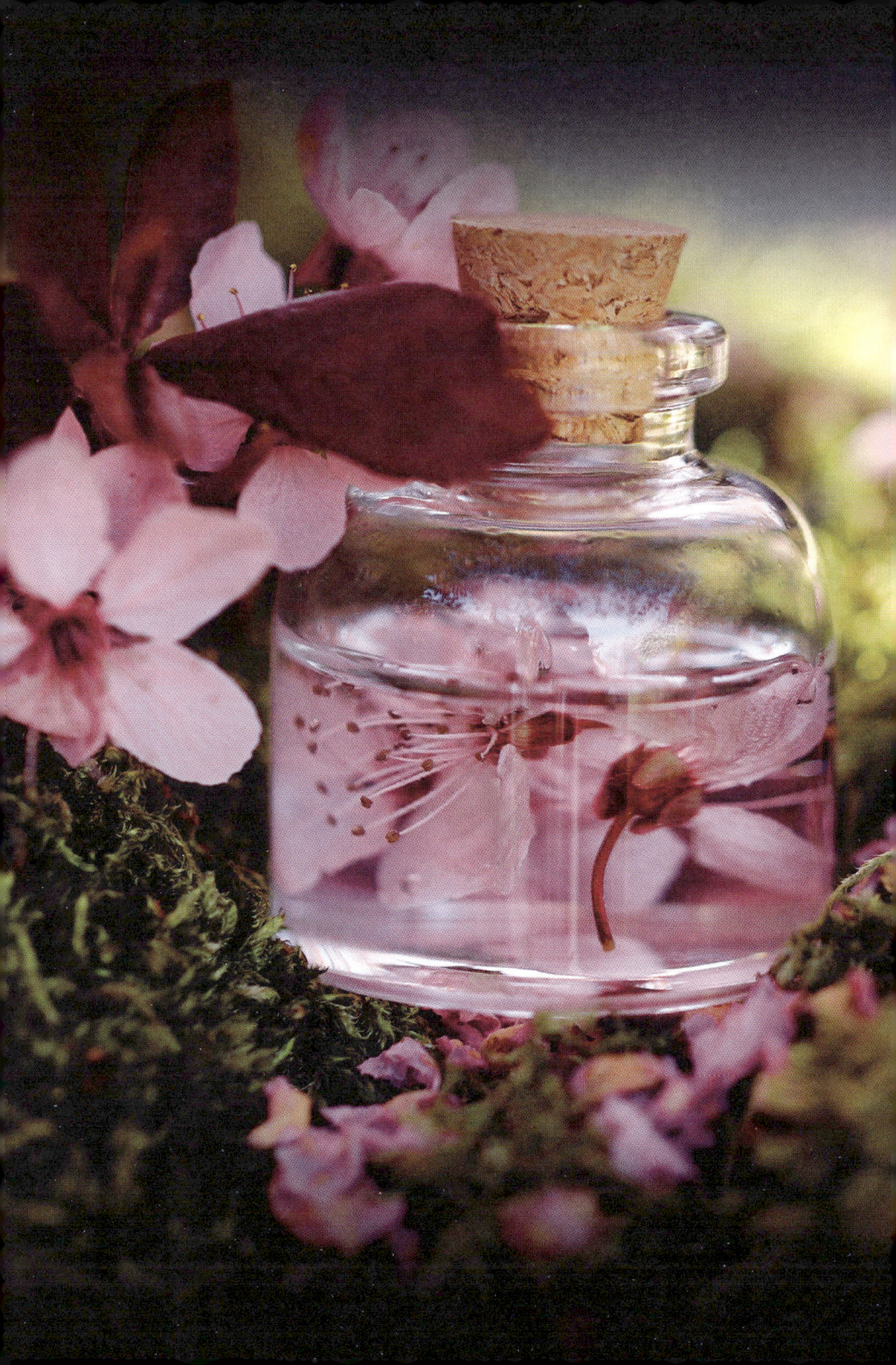

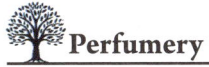

Chapter 10
Perfumery

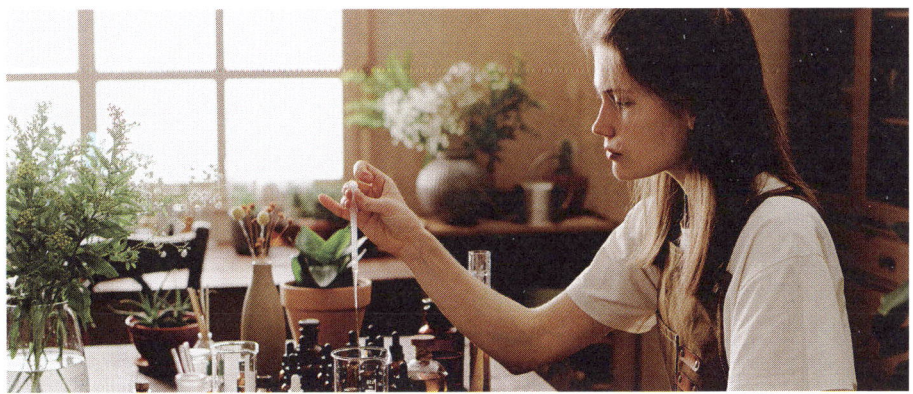

Perfumery is an art and a science. To make perfumes, one needs to know the different aromas available in synthetic and natural forms, such as essential oils. Today, many synthetic ingredients are used to make fragrances. When synthetic chemicals were not available, most body and atmosphere fragrances, including dhoops and incense sticks, were made with natural ingredients like herbs, plant materials in different forms and essential oils.

With the help of essential oils, one can make perfumes or blends that can be used as personal deodorants or to address health concerns. The advantage of essential oils is that we have access to many different oils with a variety of aromas. These can be used as perfumes with therapeutic qualities.

Let's say one is feeling dull and needs to feel energized or activate the mind and body. Then, it is advisable to make a blend of citrus oils and use it as a

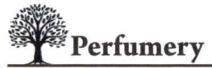 **Perfumery**

body fragrance that will lift your spirits and make you smell good. If you are experiencing stress and are deprived of proper sleep, you can make a blend with calming oils such as lavender, geranium, bergamot and a little bit of chamomile. If diffused in a room in the evenings, it will have a dual effect of infusing a pleasing aroma in the house and therapeutically will calm you and induce good sleep.

Essential oils give you different aromas along with health remedies. Reading about all the oils will make you understand the various properties but blending is a bit of an art. The best and the most trusted way of blending a perfume for yourself, especially when you require something for emotional and mental well being, is to trust your gut feeling and response. Ideally, one must have a range of essential oils in front of them. Select the oils that are therapeutically suggested for your problem. Then, smell each one; the ones you like are the ones you need to incorporate into your blend because that is what your mind

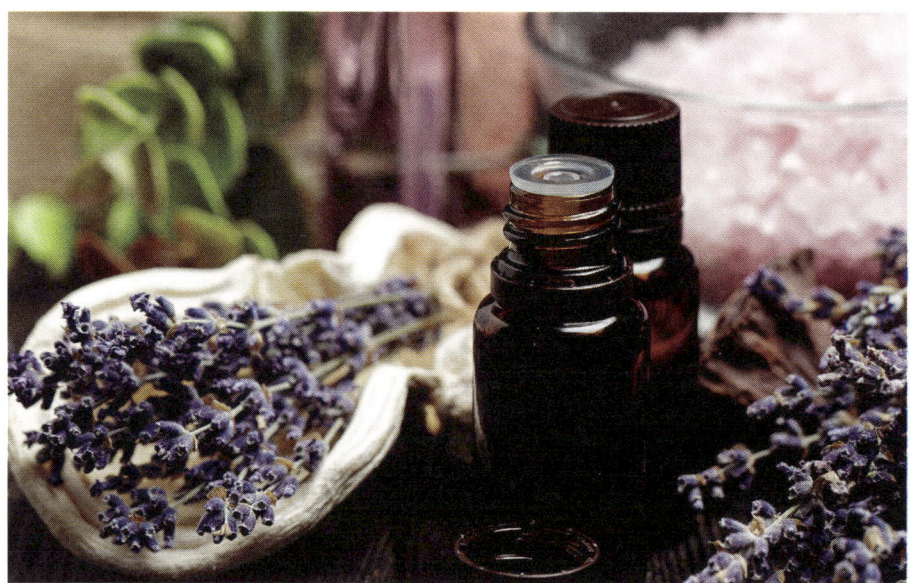

and body require. Once you have selected the oils that fit your affinity, blend them as per the notes described below.

If you like only one essential oil from the whole lot, then understand that this one is your remedy. You can use it in a diffuser, mix it with odourless alcohol and apply it to your clothes and body. You can also dilute it with a base oil and massage with it.

Let's say if your body has a deficiency of certain vitamins or minerals, your doctor asks you to take specific supplements. In the same way, the body tells you, according to the essential oil you like, that it requires that supplement to heal the imbalance. We require different essential oils to help us with issues at different times and situations. At different times of the day, specific oils can be used. It is very important to buy genuine oils to get the best results.

What are Notes?

In essential oils and perfumery, 'notes' refer to the layers of scents that unfold after a fragrance is applied. These notes-top, middle and base—are fundamental to the composition of perfumes and essential oil blends, creating a harmonious and dynamic olfactory experience.

Top Notes

Top notes, or head notes, are the initial scents that greet the nose upon application. They are light, fresh and volatile; evaporating quickly but making a significant first impression. Many top notes, such as lemon, grapefruit, eucalyptus and bergamot, have antiviral properties and add brightness to the blend. These notes are often described as sharp and assertive, quickly capturing attention and setting the stage for the fragrance's development. The fleeting nature of top notes means they usually last only a few minutes to a half-hour.

Middle Notes

Middle notes, or heart notes, last longer and provide a balancing effect. They emerge as the top notes fade, offering aromatic fullness and complexity. These notes often include floral, herbal and spice aromas that form the heart of the fragrance. They help to smooth the transition between the bright top notes and the deeper base notes, typically lasting from a few minutes to an hour or more.

Base Notes

Base notes are the final, lingering deep scents that remain after the top and middle notes have dissipated. They are rich, deep and long-lasting, grounding the blend and providing a lasting foundation for the fragrance. Base notes often come from woods, resins and roots and can linger on the skin for several hours.

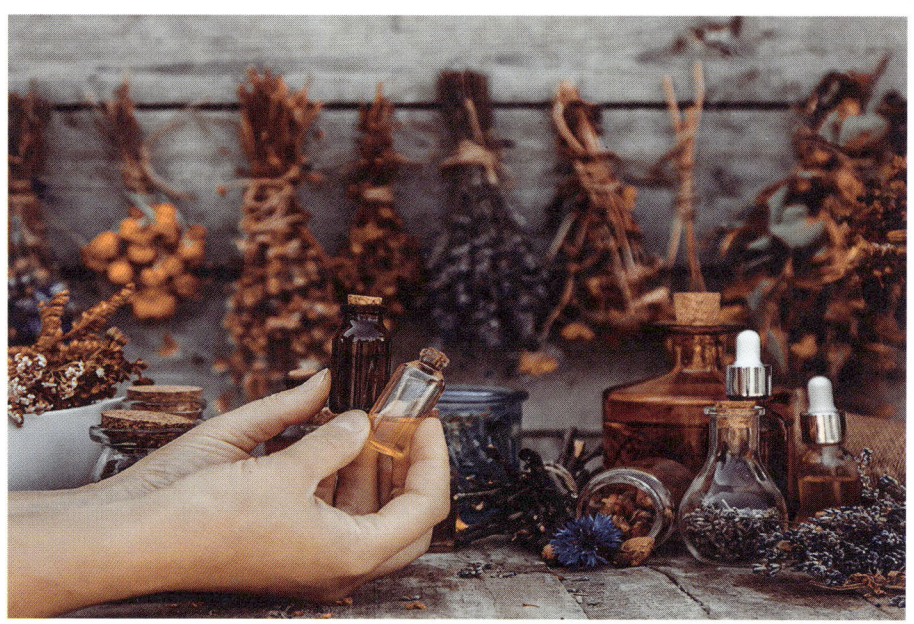

Blending Ratios

A popular blending ratio for creating balanced and harmonious essential oil blends is 3:5:2, consisting of three parts top-note oils, five parts middle-note oils and two parts base-note oils. This ratio ensures that each layer of the fragrance is represented, creating a well-rounded and dynamic blend. Adjusting the ratio can alter the overall character of the blend, allowing for customization based on personal preference or the desired therapeutic effect. Understanding the concept of notes in aromatherapy and perfumery allows for creating complex and layered fragrance experiences. Each type of note plays a crucial role in the overall scent profile, contributing to the blend's initial impression, core identity and lasting memory. Whether for therapeutic use, emotional well-being, or simply enjoying pleasant aromas, mastering the art of blending essential oils using top, middle and base notes is key to crafting effective and enjoyable aromatic experiences.

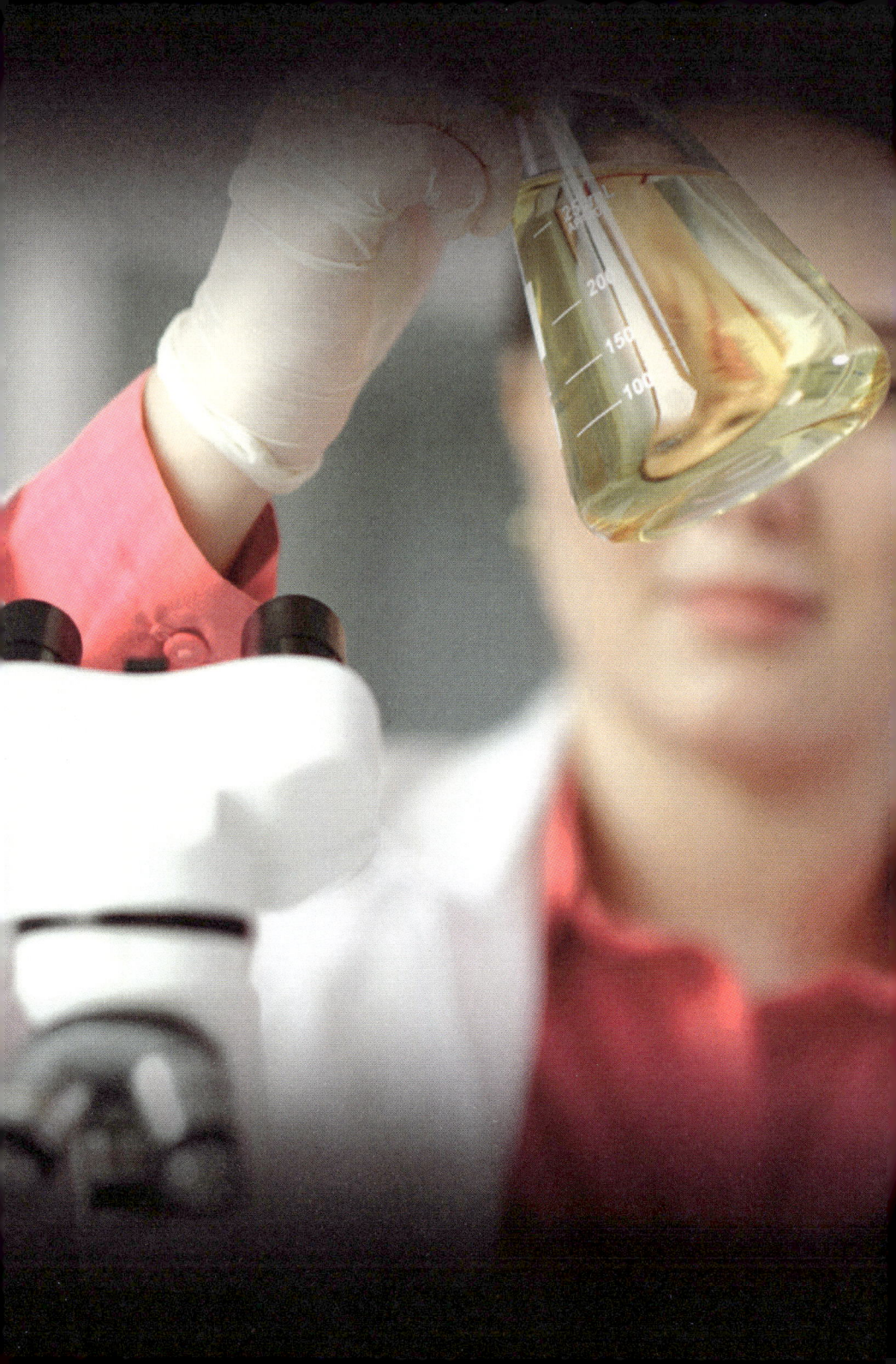

Chapter 11
Aromatherapy Blend Formulas

1. Respiratory Problems/Cold/Congestion/Viral

Essential Oils	To make 1 teaspoon of blended oil	To make 50 ml of blended oil
Eucalyptus	1 drop	7 drops
Ginger	1 drop	5 drops
Cedarwood	1 drop	7 drops
Tea Tree	1 drop	7 drops
Base Oil	To be added only in case of application	
Sesame (Til)	1 teaspoon	50 ml

Methods of Use:

1. Vaporization
2. Tissue
3. Bath
4. Apply on the chest and sinus area

2. Muscular Aches/Sprains/Arthritis/Rheumatism

Essential Oils	To make 1 teaspoon of blended oil	To make 50 ml of blended oil
Black Pepper	1 drop	4 drops
Eucalyptus	1 drop	8 drops
Ginger	1 drop	7 drops
Camphor	1 drop	6 drops
Base Oil		
Sesame (Til)	1 teaspoon	50 ml

Methods of Use:

Apply on the affected area (Do not massage)

3. Abdominal Cramps/Gas

Essential Oils	To make 1 teaspoon of blended oil	To make 50 ml of blended oil
Cumin Seed	1 drop	8 drops
Ajowan	1 drop	6 drops
Fennel Seed	1 drop	8 drops
Ginger	1 drop	7 drops
Base Oil		
Sesame (Til)	1 teaspoon	50 ml

Methods of Use:

Apply on the stomach region

Aromatherapy Blend Formulas

4. Premenstrual Syndrome

Essential Oils	To make 1 teaspoon of blended oil	To make 50 ml of blended oil
Clary Sage	1 drop	8 drops
Geranium	1 drop	8 drops
Bergamot	1 drop	8 drops
Sandalwood	1 drop	6 drops
Base Oil	To be added only in case of massage	
Sesame (Til)	1 teaspoon	50 ml

Methods of Use:

1. Vaporization
2. Tissue
3. Bath
4. Massage is to be done on the abdomen, hips, and lower back, up to the backbone

Aromatherapy Blend Formulas

5. Stress

Essential Oils	To make 1 teaspoon of blended oil	To make 50 ml of blended oil
Bergamot	1 drop	8 drops
Geranium	1 drop	8 drops
Sandalwood	1 drop	6 drops
Vetiver	1 drop	8 drops
Base Oil	To be added only in case of massage	
Sesame (Til)	1 teaspoon	30 ml
Ashwagandha		10 ml
Brahmi		10 ml

Methods of Use:

1. Vaporization
2. Tissue
3. Bath
4. Apply on temples and massage on neck and shoulder area

Aromatherapy Blend Formulas

6. Depression

Essential Oils	To make 1 teaspoon of blended oil	To make 50 ml of blended oil
Basil Tulsi	1 drop	6 drops
Clary Sage	1 drop	8 drops
Jasmin	1 drop	3 drops
Ylang Ylang	1 drop	10 drops
Base Oil	To be added only in case of massage	
Sesame (Till)	1 teaspoon	45 ml
Ashwaganda		5 ml

Methods of Use:

1. Vaporization
2. Tissue
3. Bath
4. Apply on temples and massage on neck and shoulder area

Aromatherapy Blend Formulas

7. Insomnia

Essential Oils	To make 1 teaspoon of blended oil	To make 50 ml of blended oil
Vetiver	1 drop	6 drops
Spikenard	1 drop	4 drops
Lavender	1 drop	6 drops
Ylang Ylang	1 drop	6 drops
Base Oil	To be added only in case of massage	
Sesame (Til)	1 teaspoon	40 ml
Brahmi		10 ml

Methods of Use:

1. Vaporization
2. Tissue
3. Bath to be taken with the oils before going to bed
4. Apply on temples and massage on neck and shoulder area

Aromatherapy Blend Formulas

8. Hair Fall Reduction

Essential Oils	To make 1 teaspoon of blended oil	To make 50 ml of blended oil
Spikenard	1 drop	5 drops
Carrot Seed	1 drop	6 drops
Sugandh Kokila	1 drop	6 drops
Curry Leaf	1 drop	6 drops
Base Oil	To be added only in case of massage	
Sesame (Til)	1 teaspoon	45 ml
Castor		5 ml

Methods of Use:

Part your hair and apply on the scalp. Keep for at least thirty minutes before washing.

9. Dandruff

Essential Oils	To make 1 teaspoon of blended oil	To make 50 ml of blended oil
Patchouli	1 drop	6 drops
Rosemary	1 drop	6 drops
Tea Tree	1 drop	6 drops
Cedarwood	1 drop	6 drops
Base Oil		
Sesame (Til)	1 teaspoon	45 ml
Olive		5 ml

Methods of Use:

Part your hair and apply on the scalp. Keep for at least thirty minutes before washing.

10. Dry Skin

Essential Oils	To make 1 teaspoon of blended oil	To make 50 ml of blended oil
Geranium	1 drop	8 drops
Chamomile German	1 drop	6 drops
Sandalwood	1 drop	8 drops
Vetiver	1 drop	6 drops
Base Oil		
Sweet Almond	1 teaspoon	30 ml
Apricot		20 ml

Aromatherapy Blend Formulas

Methods of Use:

Apply oil on your neck and face with upward and circulatory movements.

11. Oily Skin

Essential Oils	To make 1 teaspoon of blended oil	To make 50 ml of blended oil
Lavender	1 drop	6 drops
Cedarwood	1 drop	7 drops
Rosewood	1 drop	6 drops
Patchouli	1 drop	5 drops
Base Oil		
Aloe Vera Gel	1 teaspoon	40 ml
Jojoba		10 ml

Methods of Use:

Apply oil on your neck and face with upward and circulatory movements.

12. Acne Skin

Essential Oils	To make 1 teaspoon of blended oil	To make 50 ml of blended oil
Lavender	1 drop	3 drops
Chamomile German	1 drop	4 drops
Tea Tree	1 drop	4 drops
Base Oil		
Aloe Vera Gel	1 teaspoon	50 ml

Methods of Use:

Apply on your neck and face with upward and circulatory movements.

13. Mature/Wrinkled Skin

Essential Oils	To make 1 teaspoon of blended oil	To make 50 ml of blended oil
Frankincense	1 drop	6 drops
Carrot Seed	1 drop	8 drops
Patchouli	1 drop	8 drops
Spikenard	1 drop	4 drops
Base Oil		
Apricot	1 teaspoon	40 ml
Evening Primrose		5 ml
Ashwagandha		5 ml

Methods of Use:

Apply oil on your neck and face with upward and circulatory movements.

14. Obesity/Cellulite

Essential Oils	To make 1 teaspoon of blended oil	To make 50 ml of blended oil
Fennel	1 drop	5 drops
Juniper Berry	1 drop	5 drops
Rosemary	1 drop	5 drops
Patchouli	1 drop	5 drops
Grapefruit	1 drop	5 drops
Base Oil		
Sesame (Til)	1 teaspoon	50 ml

Methods of Use:

Massage is to be done regularly in the area where reduction is required.

If any oil is unavailable, you could substitute it with any other oil mentioned in the therapeutic index for the same problem.

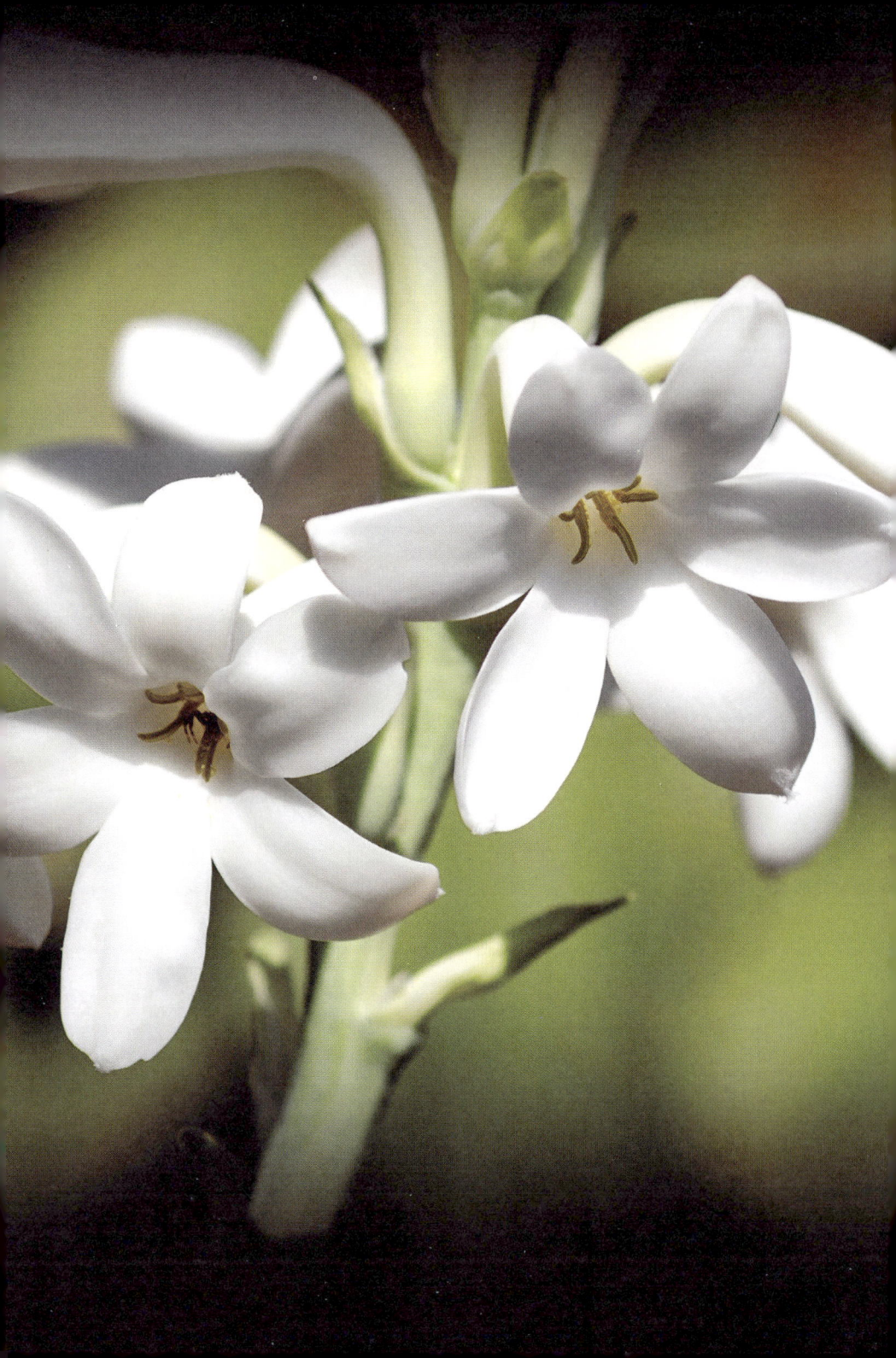

Chapter 12
Therapeutic Index For Some Common Problems

Abdominal Cramps & Gas

Basil Sweet, Bergamot, Caraway, Coriander Seed, Dill, Fennel Seed, Ajowan, Ginger, Marjoram, Peppermint, Lemongrass, Rosemary

Acne/Pimples

Cedarwood, Cajuput, Bergamot, Chamomile German, Clary Sage, Juniper Berry, Lavender, Lemon, Patchouli, Rosemary, Sandalwood, Tea Tree, Vetiver, Camphor, Palmarosa

Arthritis/Rheumatism

Black Pepper, Cajuput, Chamomile German, Chamomile Roman, Eucalyptus, Frankincense, Ginger, Juniper Berry, Marjoram, Rosemary, Camphor, Lemongrass, Nutmeg

Aphrodisiac

Clary Sage, Jasmine, Mogra, Sandalwood, Ylang Ylang

Cellulite

Cedarwood, Cypress, Fennel Seed, Lemongrass, Geranium, Patchouli, Rosemary, Basil Sweet, Juniper, Grapefruit

Therapeutic Index For Some Common Problems

Cleansing

Clary Sage, Lemon, Rosemary, Chamomile German, Lavender, Geranium, Turmeric

Cold/Flu

Tulsi, Black Pepper, Cedarwood, Eucalyptus, Ginger, Peppermint, Pine, Camphor, Tea Tree, Clove

Dandruff

Cade, Cedarwood, Clary Sage, Lemon, Patchouli, Tea Tree

Depression

Tulsi, Bergamot, Clary Sage, Geranium, Jasmine Absolute, Lavender, Petitgrain, Rose, Sandalwood, Ylang Ylang, Valerian, Mogra Absolute

Detoxification

Fennel Seed, Juniper Berry, Ravensara, Grapefruit

Dry Hair

Carrot, Cedarwood, Chamomile German, Geranium, Lavender, Palmarosa, Rosemary, Sandalwood

Eczema

Chamomile German, Frankincense, Geranium, Juniper Berry, Lavender, Patchouli, Sandalwood

Hair Loss/Fall

Bay Leaf, Carrot, Cedarwood, Curry Leaf, Palmarosa, Rosemary, Spikenard, Sugandh Kokila, Fenugreek, Cade, Clary Sage, Lemon, Patchouli

High Blood Pressure

Tulsi, Geranium, Juniper Berry, Lavender, Lemon, Marjoram, Ylang Ylang, Clary Sage

Insect Repellent

Basil Sweet, Cedarwood, Clove, Eucalyptus, Geranium, Lemon, Peppermint

Insomnia

Bergamot, Chamomile Roman, Jasmine, Lavender, Marjoram, Petitgrain, Sandalwood, Spikenard, Valerian, Vetiver, Ylang Ylang, Rose

Low Blood Pressure

Neroli, Rosemary, Thyme, Clove

Meditation

Tulsi, Frankincense, Sandalwood, Spikenard

Mental Fatigue

Basil Sweet, Cajuput, Clove, Juniper Berry, Neroli, Peppermint, Rosemary, Rosewood

PMS

Chamomile Roman, Clary Sage, Fennel Seed, Geranium, Lavender, Rose, Neroli, Sandalwood, Bergamot, Marjoram

Muscular Pain

Basil Sweet, Black Pepper, Camphor, Chamomile German, Chamomile Roman, Frankincense, Juniper Berry, Nutmeg, Marjoram, Peppermint, Rosemary, Eucalyptus, Ginger, Lemongrass

Scars

Cedarwood, Frankincense, Lavender, Myrrh, Patchouli, Carrot Seed

Skin-Combination

Geranium, Rosewood, Ylang Ylang, Palmarosa, Lavender, Sandalwood, Vetiver

For any of the above problems, use one drop each of any three to four oils mentioned and refer to the chapter on method of use.

High Blood Pressure

Tulsi, Geranium, Juniper Berry, Lavender, Lemon, Marjoram, Ylang Ylang, Clary Sage

Insect Repellent

Basil Sweet, Cedarwood, Clove, Eucalyptus, Geranium, Lemon, Peppermint

Insomnia

Bergamot, Chamomile Roman, Jasmine, Lavender, Marjoram, Petitgrain, Sandalwood, Spikenard, Valerian, Vetiver, Ylang Ylang, Rose

Low Blood Pressure

Neroli, Rosemary, Thyme, Clove

Meditation

Tulsi, Frankincense, Sandalwood, Spikenard

Mental Fatigue

Basil Sweet, Cajuput, Clove, Juniper Berry, Neroli, Peppermint, Rosemary, Rosewood

PMS

Chamomile Roman, Clary Sage, Fennel Seed, Geranium, Lavender, Rose, Neroli, Sandalwood, Bergamot, Marjoram

Muscular Pain

Basil Sweet, Black Pepper, Camphor, Chamomile German, Chamomile Roman, Frankincense, Juniper Berry, Nutmeg, Marjoram, Peppermint, Rosemary, Eucalyptus, Ginger, Lemongrass

Therapeutic Index For Some Common Problems

Scars

Cedarwood, Frankincense, Lavender, Myrrh, Patchouli, Carrot Seed

Skin-Combination

Geranium, Rosewood, Ylang Ylang, Palmarosa, Lavender, Sandalwood, Vetiver

For any of the above problems, use one drop each of any three to four oils mentioned and refer to the chapter on method of use.

About the author

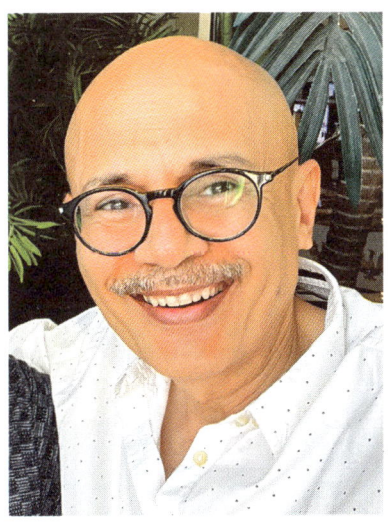

Nirmal Minawala began his journey into aromatherapy during his college years, where he gained hands-on experience in a well-equipped fragrance laboratory. The foundation of working there led him to explore various alternative healing systems using his sense of smell as guidance. He has since then found his calling in working with essential oils. Nirmal and his late wife Aradhna Minawala founded AromaTreasures, a company focused on developing high quality aromatherapy products. His work has helped provide relief for concerns such as sinusitis, joint pain, mood swings, and skin disorders.

HarperCollins *Publishers* India

At HarperCollins India, we believe in telling the best stories and finding the widest readership for our books in every format possible. We started publishing in 1992; a great deal has changed since then, but what has remained constant is the passion with which our authors write their books, the love with which readers receive them, and the sheer joy and excitement that we as publishers feel in being a part of the publishing process.

Over the years, we've had the pleasure of publishing some of the finest writing from the subcontinent and around the world, including several award-winning titles and some of the biggest bestsellers in India's publishing history. But nothing has meant more to us than the fact that millions of people have read the books we published, and that somewhere, a book of ours might have made a difference.

As we look to the future, we go back to that one word—a word which has been a driving force for us all these years.

Read.

     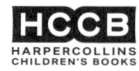

  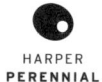   

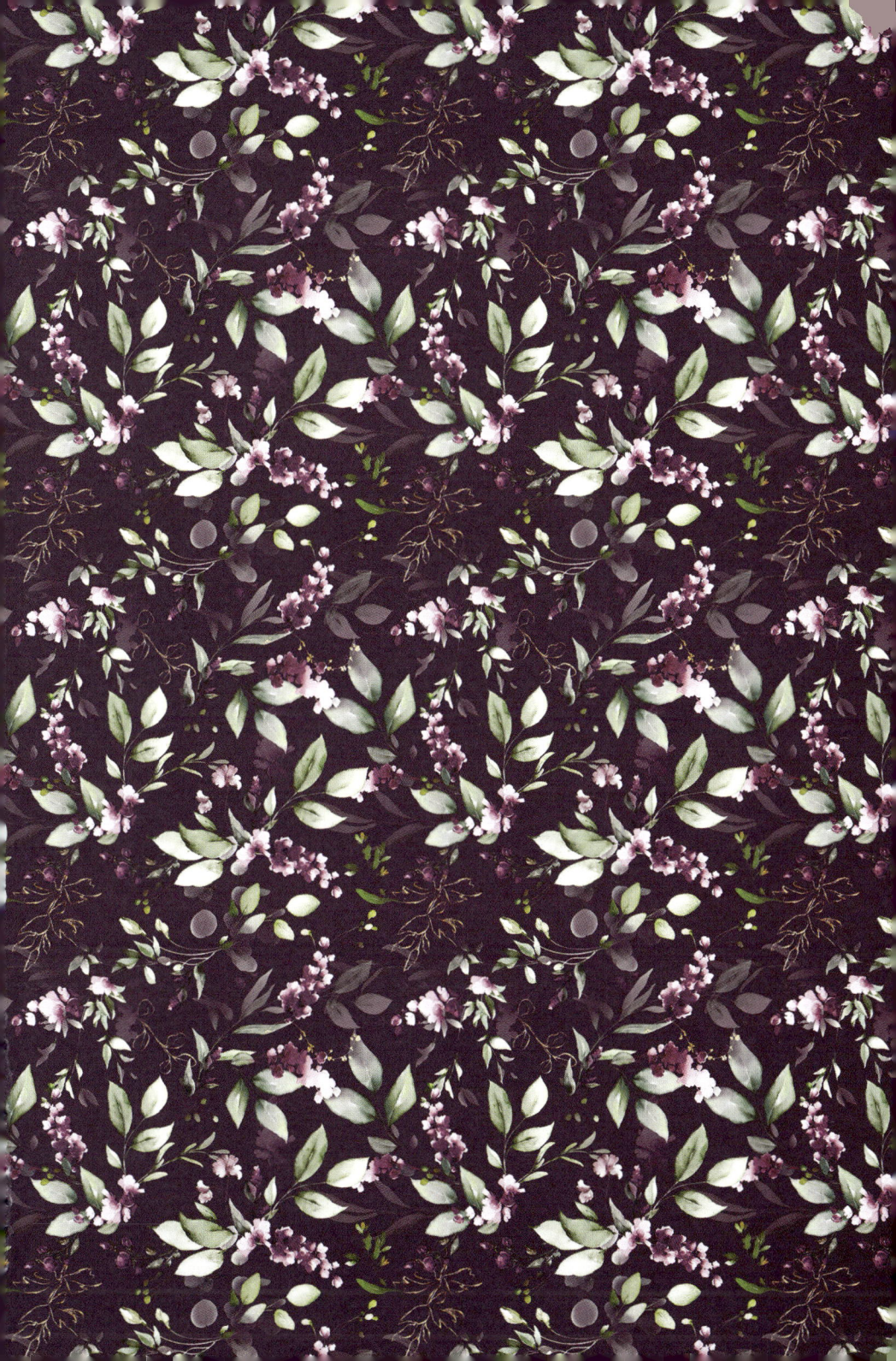

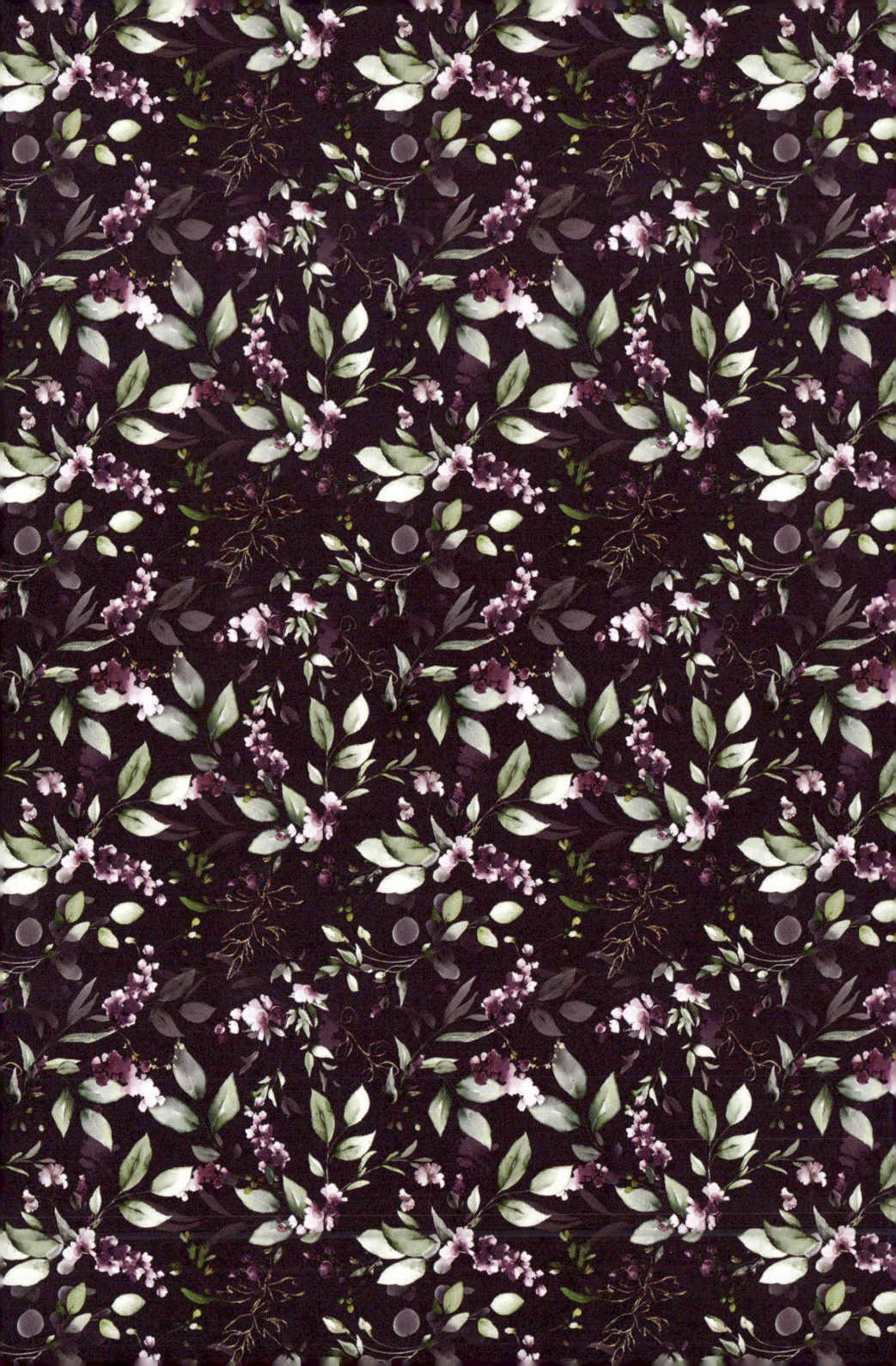